MEDICINE
with MEANING

A Doctor Discovers the
Healing Power of Homeopathy

Dr. Sandy Dinsdale

Published by My Front Door Publications, Tauranga
Contact: sandy@taurangahomeopathy.co.nz

TABLE OF CONTENTS

ACKNOWLEDGEMENTS

This book came to life through the generosity and kind support of many people. Foremost, I wish to express my gratitude to all the patients I have encountered over the years, starting from my earliest days at medical school. Their willingness to trust and share their personal stories provided the learning platform for my understanding to develop and expand, within the practice of medicine and homeopathy.

From the beginning I was fortunate to receive support from many of my homeopathic colleagues. Susanna Shelton provided encouraging feedback from the start, her characteristic enthusiasm spurring me on. I give thanks also to Gwyneth Evans, Jennie Rassell and Clive Stuart for their thoughtful input. I much appreciate the constructive comments from my GP colleagues, Dr Alison James and Dr Jackie Kamerbeek, regarding early drafts of some of the initial chapters.

I am most grateful to two dear friends, Dr Kerry Clancey and Brenda Donald, who read through the first drafts of the entire book. Their feedback was invaluable.

When my momentum stalled, I was fortunate to receive a timely boost from internationally renowned homeopath Alize Timmerman, who declared, "This book must be written!" Nearly a year later, I met Dr Robin Youngson, guest speaker at the New Zealand Council of Homeopaths AGM, who kindly shared some helpful tips on self-publishing.

My sincere appreciation goes to manuscript assessor, Jane Hole, and my editor, Daisy Coles. Their combined experience, knowledge and guidance contributed significantly to the success of this project. I also extend my appreciation to graphic designer Kerri Wheeler at Sun Media, whose expertise guaranteed the final production of a book I would be proud of.

I am grateful to Gwyneth Evans, on behalf of Julian Winston, for kind permission to use a small portion of the wealth of information contained in Julian's book, *Faces of Homeopathy* (Chapter Two). I am also thankful for kind permission given by Jan Scholten and Shambhala Publications to reproduce diagrams for this book.

On a personal note, special thanks go to my daughters, Olivia and Georgia, who graciously accepted that the dining-room table was the only practical place for their mother to write a book. I am grateful for their unwavering faith in me, and to Georgia for allowing me to share parts of her own story in this book. I much appreciate the support received from my sister, Jo Dinsdale, and from my mother, Rae Dinsdale, who expressed absolute confidence in my ability to complete this endeavour. I wish to thank Phillip Bolten for his practical assistance, and feedback regarding various design elements.

I feel most honoured and appreciative that Dr Tim Ewer, with his busy schedule as an integrative medicine physician, teacher and New Zealand board member of the Australasian Integrative Medicine Association, found time to take on the task of writing a foreword for this book.

FOREWORD

Our belief systems in medicine have changed enormously over time, and continue to do so at an accelerating pace as modern technology allows us to delve ever more deeply into the nature of our biology and the essence of life down to the quantum level. In the East, medicine derived from empirical observations of disease, and reflected the belief that our experiences, whether material, essential, or mystical, correlate with the expression of the natural order of the universe. In the West, Hippocrates is considered to be the founder of medicine as a rational science. He recognised the importance of careful observation and taking a complete history, which included environmental exposures, as well as foods eaten by the patient that might play a role in his or her illness. He believed that the goal of medicine should be to build the patient's strength and restore balance. Of particular interest to this book is his maxim "Omoia Omoiois Eisin Iamata", which translates to "like cures like".

Throughout the rapid advance of science over the last 100 years, medicine has become increasingly focused on pharmacological solutions for treating disease. Most drugs work by blocking physiological functions, and can be very effective in improving symptoms, or in killing bacteria and other micro-organisms. However, they are generally not helpful at treating the underlying cause of an illness, and tend to be better suited for acute problems rather than long-term and complex disorders. There is also the potential for a huge burden of morbidity and mortality due to the toxicity of prescription drugs (World Health Organization 2002) and the rapidly growing resistance to antibiotics (World Health Organization 2015).

More recently, there has been an increasing trend in Western society for exploring different approaches to health care, which is reflected in the large number of people (approximately 70 percent) who use complementary and alternative medicine (CAM) (Ministerial Advisory Committee of Complementary and Alternative Health, 2007). Although the reasons for this are not fully researched, it seems clear there is a growing consumer movement for greater choice, including the legitimate use of CAM (Coulter & Willis, 2004) and the role of CAM in enhancement of wellness and improved quality of life (Buettner et al., 2006). Even making time for longer consultations has been shown to directly improve health outcomes and patient satisfaction (Deveugele et al., 2002).

A New Zealand study showed that around 20 percent of general practitioners (GPs) practised one or more CAM therapies, and 32 percent had formal training in one or more CAM therapies. Almost 95 percent of GPs had referred patients to one or more CAM therapies (Poynton et al., 2006). It has been shown that patients whose GPs have additional CAM training tend to have lower healthcare costs and mortality rates (Kooreman & Baars, 2012).

Sandy Dinsdale has been generous and courageous in sharing her journey from the relative confines of general practice and reductionist medicine to the rewarding and expansive domain of homeopathy. At the heart of the healing process is the healer's willingness and ability to hold a compassionate and open space for each person's story to be fully expressed and heard. Sandy reveals how her progress into the intricacies and holistic paradigm of homeopathy has given her important tools for holding this space.

In this book, she explores the history, art and science of homeopathy, and gives a useful smorgasbord of case histories that show the wealth of her understanding and experience. The scientific bias of modern medicine is focused on randomised controlled trials (RCTs). Any system like homeopathy that sees each person's set of symptoms as highly individual and likely to require a specific remedy (which may be different to that required by another person with a medically similar diagnosis) is not going to fit easily into the RCT format. In many ways the Cartesian predominance of our scientific thinking may not be the most appropriate model for subtle methodologies like homeopathy, and the rapidly developing science of quantum mechanics may give much more insight into how ultra-low dilutions can have a therapeutic effect (Rey 2003; Tiller 2006; Ho 2011).

Sandy's use of quotations from Dr Seuss gives an added whimsical and thought-provoking nudge to challenge our habitually patterned logic, especially because that logic can so easily get in the way of openness to new concepts. As Albert Einstein said, "all the essential ideas in science were born in dramatic conflict between reality and our attempts at understanding". Einstein is also quoted as saying "the most beautiful experience we can have is the mysterious. It is the fundamental emotion which stands at the cradle of true art and true science".

Dr Tim Ewer

President of the New Zealand branch of the Australasian Integrative Medicine Association

June 2015

"I do not like green eggs and ham.
I do not like them, Sam-I-Am.

Try them, try them, and you may!
Try them and you may, I say."

Dr Seuss, *Green Eggs and Ham*

PREFACE

I had been working as a general practitioner in family medicine for ten busy years as the completion of my Diploma of Homeopathy approached, late in 2003. I recall one significant day, when I sat listening quietly in class as the history of homeopathy was recounted.

Finally I understood why doctors knew so little of its principles and practice. With a sense of responsibility I resolved to somehow make a difference; to redress the imbalance of power that had resulted in the near demise of homeopathy under the influence of a dominating medical orthodoxy.

The inspiration to write this book came some years later, with a series of personal experiences and the illness of a medical colleague.

Any residue of doubt about homeopathy as a potent messenger for change was swept away in my mind when, following completion of the Diploma, I took a homeopathic remedy in the hope of reducing monthly migraines. One of the teachers in the Diploma course had made the suggestion to me after she recalled my appreciation and affinity for the remedy themes presented in class.

I was unaware a few little white pilules would open a Pandora's box in my mind. When the key matched the lock, the lid lifted, and there was no way of closing it again, even if I'd wanted to. Within a few days I started to feel different. Uncomfortable old memories and emotions floated up, but these soon passed, leaving me with a new liberating perspective on life. There were moments of clarity in which the boundaries I'd constructed long ago lay flat, as past, present, and future became one. This experience can best be described as feeling the vast surrounding expanse of infinity while knowing oneself as a unique important part, right at the centre. It was impossible to return to my old way of being. Much grieving followed, but this was inevitable; it would've come later, if not sooner.

One day a cartoon openly dismissive of homeopathy featured in my local District Health Board's electronic newsletter. Soon after, I attended two medical education meetings presented by specialist doctors from the hospital. Both made glib negative comments about homeopathy. On both occasions I sat silently, wondering if anyone noticed my cheeks were burning, or if anyone even cared. During ten years practising homeopathy within the limitations of a busy family medical centre, I hadn't inspired one other doctor to study it, and my medical colleagues working alongside me knew little, if anything, about the homeopathic work I did. I had held long consultations with patients for chronic or recurring problems in private, and recorded these in notes that were, of course, confidential. When opportunities had arisen to offer a homeopathic remedy for an acute problem, my colleagues didn't understand the names and doses I had recorded.

The time was coming to speak up. I hoped somebody would listen.

The series of quotes from the ubiquitous Dr Seuss that found their way into this book serve as a gentle confrontation of how fixed in our thinking we become as adults, and to remind us of the curious child within us, who may yet be open to new or different ways of seeing the world.

In the beginning of the process of writing this book, I set out to inform doctors and health professionals – those with little or no knowledge of homeopathy – because these were the people I wanted to have a conversation with. I found talking to one person at a time was inefficient, and there are so many facets to this multidimensional method of healing that demand deeper exploration.

Later, as I shared more about this project with people I came into contact with, a number of non-medical people expressed interest, and I saw an opportunity to reach the public directly. The possibility of reaching a wider audience affected my approach to the language and scope of this book, and presented me with a dilemma in the ninth chapter. I needed to present genuine cases of real peoples' illness and recovery, because the homeopathic process goes deeply into the personal meaning of symptoms. This contradicted my strongly held values around privacy and confidentiality. In the end, however, those I approached for permission to use their personal information were far more relaxed about the process than I was, and without exception willing for their stories to be included. I am most grateful for their support.

Considering a more general audience, I tried to find cases that didn't involve conditions or topics that might offend, disturb or upset potential readers. This proved impossible. Human suffering is universal, and themes of deprivation, abuse, fear and violence are hidden or suppressed in many of our lives, and those of earlier generations of our families. Typically, societal and cultural norms and expectations shape our behaviour and limit our beliefs, and the darker aspects of the human condition remain out of sight. Western minds tend to keep the shadow side concealed. The case examples I've chosen for this book reveal this shadow – but at the same time they reveal the source or substance needed to facilitate healing. In this way, homeopathy holds the potential to benefit many.

Looking back, I see that my serendipitous encounter with homeopathy set me on a journey of discovery. Along the way I've learnt so much from teachers, colleagues and – most importantly – patients, who bravely shared their stories, trusting in the healing process of the consultation. Their actions demonstrate enduring qualities of hope and faith that are fundamental to human existence and endeavour.

During the writing of this book a series of growth experiences continued to unfold for me, reminding me just how deeply the healing power of homeopathy can reach.

CHAPTER ONE

A Young Doctor Encounters Homeopathy

My Story

I completed my first year of training in general practice as a registrar in 1991. Seeking more experience, I moved on to become a long-term locum in family medicine.

I first encountered homeopathy through contact with a patient early in my career. A middle-aged woman needed a skin cancer excised from the top of her foot. After suturing the skin I expressed concerns to her about how the wound would heal, because it was under tension, in a dependent mobile part of her body. These factors increased the possibility of infection and delayed healing, which might cause the wound to open up.

Graciously she declined my offer of antibiotics, saying it didn't really seem necessary. When I asked her to return after ten days for removal of the sutures, she suggested this might be too long – perhaps she would need to come in sooner? At the follow-up appointment after a week I clearly recall the nurse with a bemused appearance telling me I had better take a look – she was glad the patient hadn't waited any longer!

The skin had grown over my tidy mattress sutures, and it wasn't going to be easy to get them out. It was obvious to both of us that the extent to which the wound had healed already was beyond normal. Surprised and very curious, I asked her what she'd been doing. "I've been taking *Arnica*," was her reply. "What's *Arnica*?" was my next question, and so the conversation went, as I heard about a homeopathic remedy. She was a student studying homeopathy. She tried to explain to me what homeopathy is: not easy, as I have come to appreciate, when the person you're explaining to has no prior knowledge of the subject.

This encounter certainly left an impression with me, but I didn't explore it further until a couple of years later. On a rest home visit I met a nurse manager who was studying homeopathy, and she told me about a college running courses right here in Tauranga. At that point, I had just moved practices, and was now working part-time. I saw an opportunity worth following up, and in 1997 I enrolled at the Bay of Plenty College of Homeopathy. I took things slowly; I was still working, and also suffering from troublesome nausea of pregnancy. My first baby was due in August that year.

By some remarkable coincidence, there were two other general practitioners in my class, and we were all pregnant. Clearly we had things in common!

Curiosity and an open-minded attitude, along with a measure of scepticism and objectivity inherent in medically trained people, were other aspects I shared with the two doctors. Not infrequently, the question, "Do you really think it works?" would arise for one of us, leading to hushed but lively discussions and debates. Cautious by nature, I wasn't entirely convinced about the effectiveness of homeopathy until much later.

As doctors we were exempt from the medical science part of the training; this allowed us to focus entirely on homeopathic medicine. At the conclusion of the first year I was pleased to receive the Foundation Certificate in Homeopathy. However, I was unable to continue at that time, due to work and family commitments.

The first year of homeopathy study aims to bestow understanding and a sense of safety in prescribing remedies for *acute conditions*, including first aid and self-limiting conditions. After I had completed it, I began cautiously using remedies, mostly for myself and my family. I found homeopathic treatment for nausea in pregnancy to be effective; it preserved my sanity during a very difficult time. I had discovered I was one of those few people unable to tolerate a commonly prescribed anti-nausea medication. I made the mistake of taking a dose before stepping onto a plane. Wondering why I felt so strange, agitated and restless on the flight, I finally realised it was the medication. No way was I willing to take any more! I consulted a homeopath about "morning sickness", which in my case unfortunately lasted all day and all night. It was a great relief to me to experience a remarkable improvement in my symptoms.

Everyday life provided me with opportunities to experiment with homeopathic remedies for myself in acute situations. I recall once being utterly miserable from a slowly enlarging mouth ulcer inside my cheek. Perhaps it had started with a small trauma; I wasn't really sure. The pain was getting worse, the glands in my throat were tender, and it hurt to swallow. Painkillers didn't help. At work I discreetly resorted to rinsing a solution of steroid medicine around my mouth, which didn't relieve the pain.

Around that time, my children were becoming excited about a special school picnic being planned. The evening of the picnic, in desperation, I considered which homeopathic remedy might help, according to my symptoms. In the mirror I saw a large angry-looking ulcer completely surrounding the parotid duct, now just visible as a small dot near the centre. I pulled out a reference book listing homeopathic remedies for particular symptoms, *Kent's Repertory*, and looked up "MOUTH: Apthae". Ninety remedies were listed; too many to choose from. I moved on to "ULCERS: yellow: orifice of salivary glands, at". Three remedies were listed. I chose the one in bold type, also listed in the rubric above: *Mercurius solubis* (quicksilver). Thankfully, I had some in my bag of acute remedies. I tipped a couple of pilules into my mouth and reluctantly went on the outing as planned. When the time came to serve dinner on the school field a short while later, I realised the pain had completely gone. It never returned, and the ulcer healed. It felt like a small miracle.

A personal experience with the remedy *Opium* increased my growing interest still further. After undergoing a surgical procedure requiring a brief general anaesthetic, days later I was still lying around feeling sleepy and lethargic. My memory was terrible; I couldn't think or concentrate. My peristaltic action had completely stopped, and I was rather constipated. When things hadn't improved after a full week, I knew something was wrong, but from a medical perspective there wasn't any solution to this narcosis, apart from waiting and seeing. I had heard about the use of homeopathic *Opium* for treating the after-effects of narcotics and anaesthesia, so I rather non-committally took a dose and quickly forgot about it! The memorable part occurred a little later when, as if I'd been under hypnosis, I suddenly felt as if someone had just clicked their fingers and said, "Wake up!" At that moment I did indeed simply "wake up", and all my other symptoms soon resolved.

I returned to study homeopathy in 2001, and finally completed the Diploma of Homeopathy in 2003. At the time I felt as if I was leading a double life, practising orthodox medicine in general practice, and studying homeopathic medicine in my own time. At this point, talking about or offering homeopathic remedies at work still felt awkward to me (and possibly unethical: the vast majority of New Zealand doctors won't validate homeopathy). Now, the opposite is true, and I find it extremely difficult to remain silent about homeopathic options for treatment in my work in orthodox medicine.

The later years of the homeopathy course provided students with opportunities for clinical experience by observing and taking part in *chronic* case taking. The word "chronic" in this context refers to long-standing or recurring problems, for which patients require a deeper assessment. This involves the practitioner sitting down with the patient to hear their full story, which will reveal what remedy is needed: often referred to as the *constitutional* homeopathic remedy.

Understanding and exploring patients' stories had formed a major portion of the Royal New Zealand College of General Practice's vocational training programme that I had undertaken years before as a registrar. In 1991, our group in Dunedin was the second to experience the "Whole Person Course" facilitated by Dr Pat Farry. We began the course by telling our own stories to the group, to understand first-hand how the whole context of a person's life influences their expression of illness. This was a powerful learning experience for me.

The first chronic case I was involved in during my homeopathic training concerned a twelve-year-old boy who happened to already be registered at my general practice. One of the homeopathy teachers took the consultation, while we students watched via closed circuit television. Together we analysed his case, involving a persistent headache, and chose his remedy. However, there was no improvement, and a few weeks later his mother asked me to take the case as part of my clinical homeopathic training.

Until that point I'd only analysed "cured cases", presented on paper, to practise applying the classical homeopathic method to discover the remedy. Much to my amazement and relief, the remedy I chose and prescribed this time resulted in complete resolution of the boy's headaches.

However, I was still sceptical. Was it placebo effect? But the placebo effect apparently hadn't worked with the other homeopathic remedy the boy had been given. Maybe, I started to believe, homeopathy *did* work when the correct remedy – the *simillimum* – was discovered.

The three principles of homeopathy

The first – main – principle is "like cures like". This is a translation of the words "similia similibus curentur", and refers to a principle first observed by Hippocrates, and later by Paracelsus. In homeopathy, the remedy that works to "cure" the symptoms and/or the disease is called the *simillimum*, meaning the remedy that most similarly matches the patient's symptom picture or case. *Homos*, meaning similar, and *pathos*, meaning suffering, form the word homeopathy. The idea behind this main principle is essentially the opposite of *allopathy*, or orthodox medicine, in which a medicine is chosen for properties that work *against* the symptoms or disease. Typical examples are medicines with "anti" in their name, such as antibiotics, antivirals, antidepressants and antihypertensives. This complete contrast from the way medicine usually treats illness forms homeopathy's first challenge to the orthodox way of thinking.

The second principle of homeopathy (and challenge to the orthodox mindset) is the law of the *minimum dose*, referring to homeopathy's diluted medicines, which are not usually repeated with the same standard regularity as allopathic medicines. Homeopathic medicines undergo *potentisation*, referring to a process of serial dilution with water/alcohol alternating with vigorous shaking, called *succussion*. Succussion ensures that the healing properties of an original substance are transferred with the water/alcohol mix at each stage, making potentially poisonous substances safe to ingest. At this point in their learning about homeopathy, many people switch off or turn a blind eye; the concept seems too implausible. The challenge to their way of thinking is just too big.

I too have been challenged by homeopathy being different – but I chose to look closer, and I invite you to do the same.

The third principle of homeopathy is *individualisation*: completely individualised treatment for unique individuals. This means homeopathy only works well when the right remedy is chosen and given at the right time, in the right potency or dose. This also represents a completely different approach to conventional evidence-based medicine (EBM), where the disease rather than the person dictates the appropriate treatment.

Homeopathy and EBM: side by side

Allopathic EBM uses many algorithms to formulate proven treatments of different diseases, based on population studies. These methods result in a range of statistically predictable outcomes for disease prevention, cure or palliation, along with various side effects and adverse effects. We know it works, and we wouldn't want to be without it. I'm not suggesting homeopathy should replace the medicine we currently have. The difficulty with EBM lies in cases where outcomes are unpredictable, where people just can't tolerate the side effects, or where the risks of the standard therapies are just too high. Many disorders don't have reliable proven treatments. Medicine for the most, or for the masses, doesn't always suit the individual – or it doesn't go far enough to create health.

I don't believe there's a simple choice between allopathic medicine, including surgery, *or* homeopathic treatment – we need both. I think that the ideal is that both be used safely alongside each other. The term "alternative medicine" implies we must choose one or the other. "Complementary medicine" presents the situation more accurately, I think. On one side, EBM for many people that helps most people; on the other side, a completely individualised form of treatment. Why not choose the best of both worlds?

I've often encountered a certain illogical, rather simplistic idea within orthodox medicine: that homeopathy must be ineffective because it's not consistent with our knowledge of how allopathic medicine works. The error is in thinking these two methods can't co-exist, or that one disproves the other.

My own experience serves as example. On first reading about homeopathy, I found the concept so incongruous with what I was learning that, quite literally, I shelved it. Many years ago, while on holiday in my early medical school days, I bought a small book titled *Homeopathy: An Introductory Guide*, written in 1982 by a retired English doctor, A. C. G. Ross. Partway through the book I returned to medical school, and the overwhelming task of mastering clinical pharmacology for end-of-year exams. Spending hours in the library, I noticed no books about homeopathy. There was nothing at the medical bookshop down the road either. I assumed it must all be nonsense because none of the lecturers had mentioned it and they, of course, would know. I tossed the little book aside, closed my mind, and returned to my study.

Somehow I completely forgot about the book until I came across it again years later, when I was moving the contents of a bookcase. I didn't recall buying it until I discovered my name written inside the cover in familiar handwriting and saw a stamp from the shop where it had been purchased. At this time I was enrolled at the Bay of Plenty College of Homeopathy, and living in the same seaside town where I had bought the book.

At the opposite extreme from the exclusive EBM advocates is a group of people who only believe in homeopathy or another complementary therapy, and treat all modern allopathic medicine with fear and suspicion. This group seems to apply a similar form of illogical thinking: that both systems can't co-exist in their appropriate place. This results in a total rejection of orthodox medicine and all the benefits it has to offer.

With my experience in both homeopathy and orthodox medicine, I hope to facilitate improved awareness, tolerance and understanding of both points of view.

Homeopathy is effective, but undeniably different to allopathic EBM. It is individualised, so it can't easily be studied under the same methods as allopathy, with large double-blind randomised controlled trials. Some studies have looked at homeopathic remedies from a therapeutic perspective, basing research on remedies that might commonly be prescribed for a certain condition – but this goes against homeopathic principles, so it's far from ideal.

In spite of the apparent difficulties involved with research methods, there *is* evidence for the effectiveness of homeopathy. The New Zealand Council of Homeopaths is our regulating representative body, and their website, www.homeopathy.co.nz, has links to information.

Homeopathy in the press

The New Zealand Council of Homeopaths is occasionally called upon to respond to inaccuracies in media reports or magazine articles, and tries to balance these with accurate information. There's potential for bias when researchers set out attempting to prove that homeopathy is ineffective. A recent example occurred in a *North & South* magazine article in July 2012. The article, titled "Homeopathy – Trick or Treatment?" (Anyan, 2012), contained two key statements that are both untrue: "homeopathic remedies have failed every randomised, evidence-based scientific study seeking to verify their claims of healing powers" and "there is no scientific evidence of homeopathy's efficacy".

A formal complaint was laid with the New Zealand Press Council, "that the article and accompanying editorial were highly derogatory, inaccurate and misleading". The complaint was upheld.

Similarly, an article published in the *New Zealand Listener* some years ago caused considerable harm to homeopathy. Relaxing in the sun on the local beach, my surprise at finding an article in this widely read magazine about the homeopathic remedy *Arnica* soon turned to dismay. The study quoted had apparently found that *Arnica* was not effective in treating the condition carpal tunnel syndrome. My peaceful relaxation was shattered as I realised this respected magazine would be read by thousands of people who would be influenced by the apparent disproval. Sadly, I still encounter some of those people, who refer to the article they read in good faith years earlier.

To test a homeopathic remedy in the same way as a therapy for a particular therapeutic condition is methodologically flawed, but to test it against a condition that's unlikely to indicate *Arnica* as a remedy is simply wrong. This study clearly wasn't designed by homeopaths. At best, it was ignorant of homeopathic principles; at worst, it was sabotage. Trialling *Arnica* to treat carpal tunnel syndrome is akin to trialling aspirin to treat depression. If aspirin was shown not to be effective in such a trial, so what? Would this mean aspirin was ineffective in all circumstances? Could we then extrapolate the findings to say that all allopathic medicine is ineffective? Letters to the editor from homeopaths were published in later editions of the magazine, but the damage was already done.

These examples illustrate a long-standing division between orthodox and homeopathic medicine. It's time for a change in our thinking; time to move forward. But first we need to understand how this split occurred, to fully comprehend why homeopathy remains unrecognised and underutilised in current medical practice in New Zealand, and much of the Western world.

CHAPTER TWO

A Brief History of Homeopathy

Homeopathy's beginnings

No book about homeopathy would be complete without reference to the origins of this remarkable healing method.

German physician Samuel Hahnemann is credited with discovering and developing homeopathy in 1790. Historically, both Hippocrates and Paracelsus were already known to have suggested that "like cures like", but Hahnemann took the concept to a new level.

Homeopathic historian Julian Winston published *The Faces of Homeopathy: an Illustrated History of the First 200 Years* in 1999. The book is meticulously researched, and includes photographs and information never previously published. In Winston's own words, *"Faces of Homeopathy* is the first book to tell the whole story – from Hahnemann through the contemporary homeopaths in the 1990s". In recounting some of the early history of homeopathy, I have drawn from this text.

Philosophically speaking, homeopathy originated during the Age of Enlightenment.

Samuel Hahnemann and the *Cinchona* experiment

Samuel Hahnemann (1755–1843) completed his medical degree in 1779 at the University of Leipzig, in Germany. As a student, he had earned extra income using his linguistic talent to translate books from English into German. While translating a medical book by Dr William Cullen, he became interested in the relationship between the curative effects of *Cinchona* from the Peruvian bark tree (*Cinchona officinalis*, also known as China) and its poisoning symptoms. He observed close similarity between the symptoms already known to result from poisoning by *Cinchona* (cinchonism), and those of the intermittent fever it was commonly used to treat. Historical evidence indicates that Hahnemann took cinchona bark himself to test this theory, as he wrote a footnote in Cullen's book, *A Treatise of the Materia Medica*, describing his experience:

> I took, for several days, as an experiment, four drams of good China twice daily. My feet and finger tips, etc at first became cold. I became languid and drowsy; then my heart began to palpate; my pulse became hard and quick; an intolerable anxiety and trembling (but without a rigor); prostration in all the limbs; then pulsations in the head, redness of the cheeks, thirst . . . all those symptoms which are typical of intermittent fever. . . This paroxysm lasted for two to three hours every time, and recurred when I repeated the dose, and not otherwise. I discontinued the medicine and I was once more in good health. (Winston, 1999, p. 4)

The concept that a substance used to treat a disease caused similar symptoms to that disease, and that this might be the reason why *Cinchona* was effective in treating intermittent fever, was not yet known. This concept forms the basis of the "Law of Similars" in homeopathy. The process Hahnemann used – taking small doses of a substance and noting the effects – is still used today as a way of *proving* a homeopathic remedy. Hahnemann went on to prove 106 homeopathic remedies during his lifetime.

We know Hahnemann was disillusioned with the ineffectiveness and the potential to cause further harm of the medicine he saw practised around him. He was interested in the benefits of a healthy diet and non-interventionist treatments. In 1792 he spoke against popular treatments of the day that were harmful, including blood-letting. Emperor Leopold II of Austria had recently tragically bled to death as a result of this practice. In 1796 Hahnemann published his ideas in his "Essay on a New Principle for Ascertaining the Curative Powers of Drugs, and Some Examination of the Previous Principles". A few years later he started practising clinical medicine again, applying this new methodology.

Later Hahnemann wrote more about the provings in his book *Materia Medica Pura* (1821). He later published another book, *Chronic Diseases* (1828), which he had written while maintaining a now busy homeopathic practice.

Hahnemann's early development of homeopathy occurred during a time when allopathic medicine wasn't particularly effective, and was sometimes harmful. It might be argued that this alone was the reason for its early success. However, the historical statistics indicate otherwise. During a typhus outbreak in 1813 during the Battle of Leipzig, at the time of Napoleon's retreat from Moscow, Hahnemann documented cured cases totalling 178 out of 180 people he treated, in comparison to a mortality rate among those treated allopathically of 20–30 percent. Homeopathy is also credited with curing many cases of cholera during the European epidemic of 1831–1832.

At age seventy-nine Hahnemann was married for the second time, to Melanie D'Hervilly, a woman in her thirties who had travelled alone from Paris to Germany just to meet him. She'd lost friends to the cholera epidemic, and had witnessed people receiving successful homeopathic treatment by a local doctor. After reading one of Hahnemann's publications, *Organon of Medicine*, Melanie was determined to pay Hahnemann a visit. By all accounts, she was a remarkable woman. Her liberal upbringing allowed her to enjoy more freedom than many women during this period. She found that she could travel more safely dressed as a man, and reportedly said, "I prefer going about with men, for no sensible word can be addressed to a woman!"

Melanie became a pupil of Hahnemann, and practised homeopathy under his oversight. The two moved to Paris in 1835. Among their patients there were some of the famous and elite, including the musician Paganini and the writer Balzac.

After a long and productive life, Samuel Hahnemann died in 1843 at age eighty-eight, following a chest infection. A year earlier, he'd completed the sixth edition of the *Organon*, which remained unpublished until 1920. This edition is still widely used today.

Homeopathy comes to the United States

Homeopathy spread from Germany to the United States. It was practised in America as early as the 1820s by some who had learnt directly from Hahnemann's followers.

Constantine Hering was a German-born practitioner who went on to become a significant figure within the discipline. Like so many who followed, he developed an interest in homeopathy after a personal curative experience. His right index finger was wounded in 1821, and he declined to undergo the treatment of the day, which was amputation. A friend suggested he take a minute dose of *Arsenicum* (arsenic). He did so, and after consequently recovering from the wound without the need for surgery, he began corresponding with Hahnemann. Hering graduated as a doctor 1826, and undertook the first "proving" of *Lachesis*, the homeopathic remedy made from a bushmaster snake, in 1828. It's reported that he stunned the snake with a blow to the head, and then milked the venom himself to make the remedy. Hering moved to the United States in 1833, and there helped open the first homeopathic school in the world. He is famous for "Hering's Law of Cure", describing the usual sequence or direction of improvement in a patient's symptoms during successful homeopathic treatment.

Other early practitioners were drawn to homeopathy after experiencing the results of treatment first-hand. Claude Boenninghausen was one such. He never became a medical doctor, but wrote the first homeopathic repertory in 1832. He had fallen ill with tuberculosis in 1827, and, believing that death was inevitable, wrote farewell letters to his friends. One friend, who knew about homeopathy, wrote back to him, to obtain a more detailed understanding of his symptoms. The friend then sent Boenninghausen a well-chosen homeopathic remedy, and after a few months he recovered. Boenninghausen's Repertory remains in use today.

(Repertories are books indexed by symptoms listing particular remedies known to cause or reproduce a specific symptom. Materia medica are essentially the opposite: indexed by remedy, they describe the symptoms noted in provings, accidental poisonings and successfully "cured" cases. Homeopaths use repertories and materia medica as tools to select and confirm the simillimum.)

Homeopathy spread by virtue of its reputation, and as more and more medical doctors began to turn to homeopathy, the discipline began to represent a threat to orthodox medicine. Perhaps a backlash was inevitable.

Arguably the first significant reaction from the orthodox medical community was that which had followed soon after Samuel Hahnemann published his first article about the principle of "similars" in medicine.

Rival institutes

A group of homeopaths founded the American Institute of Homeopathy in 1844 in response to their perception of a lack of national medical standards. Their aim was to further develop homeopathy and to improve the quality of medicine practised. Just three years later, the American Medical Association (AMA) formed in open opposition, creating a significant historical division. The American Medical Association's membership contract contained a clause preventing any member from consulting with any other practitioner "whose practice is based on an exclusive dogma to the rejection of the accumulated experience of the profession". Effectively, this meant any doctor could be expelled from the AMA if they even spoke to a homeopath.

Within a few years, all formal communication between the two branches of the medical profession stopped. Allopathic doctors were prevented by their membership in the AMA from buying medicines from homeopathic pharmacies, and medical schools could refuse entry to anyone sympathetic to homeopathy. Moreover, the schools could prevent any of their students who even had an interest in homeopathy from sitting their final examinations.

The purging of homeopathy by the allopathic community effectively forced homeopaths out of medical practice. It seems likely that further development of homeopathic medicine was weakened by this process. Remarkably, however, in spite of this division, over twenty homeopathic medical colleges were formed in America over the next few years, set up by medical doctors who had adopted homeopathy.

The influenza pandemic of 1918 was a worldwide tragedy: resulting mortality is estimated at 20 million people. At the time, homeopathic doctors in the United States recorded mortality rates for the influenza among their patients of around 1 percent. Their treatment mostly comprised two well-known remedies, *Gelsemium* and *Bryonia*. In contrast, the mortality rate for patients treated with allopathic medicine was 30 percent. In this case, treatment mostly involved salicylic acid and some quinine in material doses.

The birth of pharmaceuticals

The next challenge to homeopathy came when pharmaceutical companies started up to supply medicines during the American Civil War. Previously, most medicines had been obtained from plant sources; information about their effects had come from traditional and homeopathic use. A trend emerged for manufacturing "patent" proprietary medicines, using a formulation known only to the pharmaceutical company. The AMA banned medicines using such secret formulations for ethical reasons, but the ban was sidestepped by the manufacturers of proprietary products who claimed that the formulas they marketed under their individual trade names were subject to copyright. Drug advertisements in the *Journal of the American Medical Association* listed ingredients without printing the actual formula.

This was the beginning of an enduring close relationship between pharmaceutical companies and allopathic medicine. The financial contributions of such companies continue to influence the direction of medicine, and the two remain closely linked. In contrast, homeopathic remedies are not secret or subject to patent. Information about the contents and potency of remedies are not owned by any one individual or group. Proving and therapeutic information is shared through publication, and methods of manufacture have remained largely unchanged. They are standardised and relatively simple, as laid out in the *Homeopathic Pharmacopoeia* (the Homeopathic Pharmacopoeia of the United States has been in continuous publication since 1897; it is now published online).

Homeopathy spreads to England

Homeopathy began to gain popularity in England around the same time it spread to the United States from Germany. There were many successful homeopathic medical schools and hospitals in England during the later 1800s.

In England, the royal family have traditionally been supporters of homeopathy. Like many others, royal physician Sir John Weir (1879–1971), who treated the family (including the current queen) from 1918 until he retired in 1968, learnt about homeopathy from a colleague who treated him effectively with this type of medicine. Dr Margery Blackie took over Weir's role, followed in 1980 by Dr Peter Fisher, medical director of the Royal London Homeopathic Hospital. Queen Elizabeth II remains the patron of this famous hospital.

In the early 1900s, a mechanistic view of the human body as a machine with various interacting parts emerged; this still forms the basis of "modern medicine". The process of investigating and understanding anatomy and physiology has undoubtedly provided much medical progress. However, homeopathy considers that a view of human illness that aims to correct abnormalities of specific parts runs the risk of losing sight of the whole person.

The emergence of the mechanistic view also began to affect the way homeopathy was taught and used. Much as allopathic medicines were used to treat a particular disease or condition, homeopathic medicines started to be prescribed in a similar way, in a method known as "therapeutics", whereby a remedy was chosen from those known to have cured others with the same condition. Most medicines prescribed in this way were herbal tinctures containing material doses to be taken repeatedly, much like allopathic medicines.

These changes went against the Law of Similars and the principle of individualisation, and threatened the survival of classical homeopathy. Homeopathy since Hahnemann's day had been about treating the whole symptom picture on a mental, emotional and physical level; a concept known as the Totality of Symptoms. Illness was considered as a derangement of a person's vital force or life energy. These timeless principles are carefully recorded in the *Organon*.

The development of homeopathy occurred alongside the women's suffrage movement, and each affected the other. The first female homeopath was Hahnemann's wife Melanie, a non-medical practitioner who was later awarded an honorary diploma. In those early days, medicine was dominated by men. In the Victorian era, women were generally considered weak and prone to sickness. At the same time, it was difficult for women to receive medical care from male doctors due to the morals of the day, and they weren't allowed to enter educational institutions, so they looked to each other for help. Women were the ones to provide general care when "expert" help wasn't available, and groups of better informed women set up groups to teach others about hygiene principles.

Hering published *Domestic Physician* in 1835. It was the first homeopathic manual for home use, and came to be relied on by women in the community applying its principles to treat the poor. This book played a part in making homeopathy accessible to anyone; some of the colleges eventually accepted females during the 1850s. The American Institute of Homeopathy welcomed women members in 1870, five years before the American Medical Association allowed female medical students.

As a direct result of the historical division between orthodox medicine and homeopathy, the majority of homeopathy practitioners in recent times are non-medical.

Considering the history, it's remarkable that homeopathy is still used all over the world, including in Europe, India, South America, Africa, Australia, New Zealand and the United States.

Homeopathic remedies have a proven safety record and are relatively cheap to produce, making good economic and environmental sense. Next, we look more closely at the production of these controversial medicines, and consider how the "information" they contain might be transferred.

CHAPTER THREE

The Infinitesimal Dose

The preparation of homeopathic remedies

Homeopathic medicines are usually referred to as *remedies* to avoid any confusion with orthodox or herbal medicines. Throughout this book the word homeopathy refers to *classical homeopathy*, as originally developed and practised by Samuel Hahnemann. This can be confusing, as many other homeopathic methodologies have developed over the years, and a variety of health practitioners including homeopaths use homeopathic remedies in different ways outside the sphere of classical homeopathy.

Homeopathic remedies are made mostly from plants, minerals and animal or human tissue, which may be healthy (*sarcodes*) or diseased (*nosodes*). Strict protocols are used for their production according to the *Homeopathic Pharmacopoeia*, drawing from Hahnemann's original book, the *Organon of Medicine*.

The starting point for traditional homeopathic remedies is a small amount of either a plant tincture or insoluble substance that is *triturated*, meaning ground up using a mortar and pestle along with milk sugar (lactose powder). As a fine powder these substances become soluble in a 50/50 water and alcohol mix, and are ready for dilution.

The next stage is *serial dilution* and *potentisation* of the liquid using a method known as *succussion*, a form of vigorous mixing following each step of dilution. Most homeopathic remedies are made using a 1:100 dilution referred to as centesimal or C potency. Those made using 1:10 dilution are referred to as decimal or X potency. Succussion between each dilution is performed by banging the vial of liquid against a firm surface, a process best carried out by hand. Many doses of a remedy can be made from a small amount of the original substance, making the preparation of homeopathic medicines both environmentally friendly and economical.

After potentisation the liquid remedy can be either dispensed as liquid or soaked into pilules. Pilules consist of a plain sugar carrier that absorbs the homeopathic liquid, making administration easy and convenient. Doses are usually administered into the mouth, where they dissolve, ideally, under the tongue. Alternatively a few drops of the homeopathic remedy as a liquid can be taken in a little water and swallowed.

A remedy of a commonly used potency, 30C, has been through the process of dilution 1:100 followed by succussion a total of 30 times, resulting in a very dilute but potent solution. Homeopathic remedies can even be made from substances normally considered poisonous or harmful because they don't contain even a single molecule of the original substance. Because homeopathic remedies do not contain material doses of the original substance at all, the words *infinitesimal dose* or *ultramolecular dilution* may be used.

How do homeopathic remedies work?

At this point I've noticed my medical colleagues' eyes start glazing over, because it's completely different to allopathic medicine. How can homeopathic remedies possibly work? The answer is that we don't yet know the exact mechanism, but it's highly likely they work by a *memory* or *signature message* of the original substance being carried within the water and alcohol mixture. We do know from accumulated years of observation and experience how homeopathic remedies *behave*, and how to assess their effects in clinical use.

Many laboratory experiments have demonstrated that water can carry information from a substance dissolved in it, even at ultramolecular dilutions. The most famous of these experiments was undertaken by Dr Jacques Benveniste and a team of French scientists, who published their findings in the journal *Nature* in 1988. Benveniste was undertaking research into allergies at the time. His reputation as a biologist was already well established.

The initial indication that water could transmit such a "memory" occurred serendipitously, due to a simple error in laboratory calculation during Benveniste's research, which involved anti-IgE antibodies. By accident, the scientists ended up testing a much more dilute aqueous solution of these antibodies than they had intended. However, they found that this solution caused a similar effect to that they would have expected from a concentrated molecular solution.

As a condition of publication of Benveniste's findings, the journal *Nature* asked for his results to be replicated by independent laboratories. Experiments into the transmission of "information" (that is, the effect of anti-IgE) in ultra-dilute liquid were therefore replicated in four other laboratories in France, Canada, Israel and Italy. Researchers found that control solutions that did not contain any anti-IgE were ineffective. Further, they found that those control solutions that contained ultra-dilute anti-IgE, but that did not undergo any succussion, were less effective, showing that vigorous shaking is an important step for the transmission of "information".

Outside the sphere of homeopathy, this research has important implications for our knowledge about how information is carried between cells within living organisms. Our own bodies are made up of approximately 70 percent water; the ramifications of the discovery that water is able to transmit information between cells are far reaching.

The next step up from studying the effects of ultra-dilute solutions on isolated cells involves experimentation with organ tissues – under controlled laboratory conditions. Such experiments have been carried out with highly diluted substances, resulting in effects on the organ that were similar to what they would have been had a concentrated molecular solution been used. Benveniste himself went on to demonstrate that the injection of ultra-high dilutions of a substance capable of increasing blood flow through the coronary vessels of isolated guinea pig hearts had a similar effect to material doses (Benveniste et al., 1992).

A year or two later Benveniste and his fellow researchers took things a step further. In a new experiment, closed vials of substances capable of stimulating the hearts, and of plain water as control, were placed inside a coil through which an electric current was passed. An amplifier then delivered the current to *another* coil surrounding a closed vial of plain water. Only the water treated with current from the coils around the stimulating substances, when injected through the guinea pig heart, was able to increase coronary blood flow (Benveniste et al., 1994). They demonstrated that treated water also carried information via an electromagnetic field specific to the original substance, and that this had a similar effect on an isolated organ.

Messages in water: Masaru Emoto

Japanese researcher Masaru Emoto gained worldwide popularity upon publication of his first book, *Messages from Water*. When a colleague introduced Emoto to a type of water that worked miraculously to treat his foot pain, he had become motivated to study the *information* carried by water, and how this might affect the mind and body.

Emoto's experiments involved putting water into a glass bottle and exposing it to information such as one or two words, a picture, or music, then freezing the drops of water on petrie dishes. Under a microscope, Emoto's team saw that tiny grains of ice in this water tended to form crystals, but not always. Some dishes contained intricate beautifully formed symmetrical crystals, and others had partially formed or collapsed crystals, or sometimes none at all. The water crystals appeared to be indicative of the "quality" of water that had been studied. For example, tap water from cities with a close supply of naturally occurring water showed more complete crystal formation, and water from cities known for "poor" quality water often showed none.

Emoto found that water seemed to "understand words". When he exposed it to positive words like "happiness", it formed crystals with a balanced even shape upon freezing. In contrast, negative words like "unhappiness" resulted in broken and unbalanced crystals. The research was carried out in a variety of languages, and the responses were similar but not identical. I recommend taking a look at Masaru Emoto's books, available in many local libraries (see, for example, Emoto, 2005), to fully appreciate the extent of his work and contemplate the "messages" revealed by the photos.

Many people believe science is a long way from explaining how material substances can imprint information into water, as they do to form homeopathic remedies. However, already, arguments based on the implausibility of infinitesimal doses having any effect can be refuted by considering the *structure* of water.

The structure of water: Rustum Roy

Professor of chemistry and physics Rustum Roy, who died in 2010, left behind a legacy of work demonstrating that water is capable of effects far beyond those indicated by simple chemistry (see, for example, Roy et al., 2005).

Roy suggests that the *structure* of water, rather than its *chemical composition*, determines its properties. To illustrate, he compares the well-known carbon composition of an extremely hard diamond with that of soft graphite, also composed of carbon. These widely differing properties are the result of chemical bonds. Strong equal carbon bonds hold a diamond together rigidly; in contrast, unequal carbon bonds hold graphite together softly, so layers rub off, as when we write with a graphite pencil. Because water has highly unequal bonding, it comes in many structures with different properties. What we think of as simply "H_2O" can be changed by electromagnetic fields, pressure and *epitaxy*, which Rustum Roy defines as the transfer of information without matter; the imprinting of one structure onto another.

Roy explains that suspending an electromagnetically charged nanoparticle in water causes the water to change to become a *colloid* or *aquasol* (a fine solid particle dispersed permanently in water). He suggests that the very high pressures (10 to 15,000 atmospheres) applied to particles during the processes of trituration and succussion used to make homeopathic remedies can also change water by epitaxy forming an aquasol. Roy reminds us that water is not all the same, and is certainly not homogeneous.

Other laboratory evidence for homeopathy

Certain experiments have tested the effects of potentised homeopathic remedies on organ tissues, with significant results. For example, in 1997, Cristea et al. applied a solution of the homeopathic medicine *Belladonna* (from deadly nightshade plant) to a piece of rat intestine. At lower dilutions (1c to 20c) the smooth muscle of the intestine relaxed, while at higher dilutions (30c to 45c) it contracted. The main active substance in *Belladonna* is atropine, which is known to be capable of either increasing or decreasing the contraction of smooth muscle, depending on the level of dilution.

This brings to my mind an interesting experience I had years ago. One evening, I treated my daughter for an ear infection with *Belladonna*. Later that evening, her father picked up a pilule of it off the floor. He discarded it, then continued working at his computer. Soon after, he asked me if I would check his eyes, because he could no longer focus on the words in front of him! I knew that even handling a homeopathic remedy could sometimes result in temporary effects, and that atropine could affect the eye (atropine itself causes prolonged dilatation of the pupils). He was experiencing the *symptom* of difficulty focusing, having *proved* the remedy by holding it. I was able to reassure him the effect shouldn't last too long.

It's beyond the scope of this book to list the various research studies and evidence to date regarding homeopathy.

I encourage interested readers to look at the excellent websites of the New Zealand Council of Homeopaths and the New Zealand Homeopathic Society locally, and further abroad, those of the British Homeopathic Association, the United Kingdom Faculty of Homeopathy, and the North American Society of Homeopaths. All provide useful information, references to research, and regular updates. They also list the accumulated evidence for the effectiveness of homeopathy for many specific acute and chronic conditions.

The placebo effect

Many sceptics of homeopathy claim that its success is all due to placebo effect. Across the board (that is, in a phenomenon that applies equally to allopathic medicines, surgical treatments, and homeopathy), the placebo effect has been demonstrated to be significant: when a person *thinks* they've been treated with something helpful, their symptoms improve by up to 30 percent.

One way of testing a particular treatment without the complication of the placebo effect is to test it on animals, and indeed many studies have found positive results supporting the effectiveness of ultra-high-dilution homeopathic remedies in animals.

Testing treatments: the rationalist method

19th-century orthodox medicine was developed along rationalist lines by early practitioners Galen and Boerhaave, who believed a physician could acquire knowledge about a patient and about medicines a priori: by deduction. The rationalist method only recognises symptoms that can be connected with an assumed pathological process; these symptoms are referred to as *legitimate*. (As an aside, I prefer the modern term *bio-medical method* to refer to this method, to avoid any assumption that other methods are less than "rational".) Symptoms that are not understood and don't suit the existing theory are discounted or considered illegitimate. This supposedly establishes a cause-and-effect relationship, and is considered to be a scientific view of illness.

Nowadays, in testing orthodox medicine, randomised controlled trials (RCT) are considered to be the gold standard. This process results in what is known as *rational medical therapeutics*.

Randomised control trials operate as follows. *Randomisation* refers to the process of assigning trial subjects to either treatment or control groups, to avoid bias caused by selection (for example, subjects of a particular age or socioeconomic background being assigned to the same group; this could affect the ultimate results of the test). *Control* refers to trial subjects within a particular study who do *not* receive the treatment, to allow comparison of treated and untreated subjects – this allows for the potential effects of chance or placebo effect. Randomised control trials ideally also involve *double blinding*, which refers to a situation in which neither the person administering the treatment nor the person receiving it knows which group (treated or control) each subject belongs to.

The RCT is useful as a tool for research, but it doesn't necessarily apply to all therapeutics. I have spent some time considering the difficulties inherent in applying the RCT method to homeopathy.

Testing treatments: the empirical method

In contrast to rationalists, empiricists assume that every single symptom expressed by a person proceeds from one cause to another, without attempting to isolate causes.

Homeopathy is based on the empirical method. Historian and homeopath Harris Coulter (1932–2009) explored the history of Western medicine in a series of books, *Divided Legacy* Volumes I–IV. Coulter explains how the empirical method is based on pure observation of patients as the source of knowledge, and that this method stresses the primary importance of symptoms (Coulter, 1982).

Empiricists observe all of a patient's symptoms and all of the effects of medicines they are given. Samuel Hahnemann was an empiricist; his predecessors were Hippocrates, Paracelsus, Stahl, and the Greek Empirical School. Hahnemann went a step further than the Greeks with his idea of testing medicines by *proving* them on healthy subjects – this was highly innovative at the time. He observed a direct connection between the diagnosis or symptom picture, and treatment; this formed what became known as the Law of Similars. The direct connection between all of the symptoms *and* the therapy led Coulter to conclude that "homeopathy is based on an integrated coherent doctrine for its therapeutic practice".

I'm trained as both an allopath (a rationalist) and a homeopath (an empiricist). I can illustrate the difference with a case example from my own experience. A patient consults me with a flu-like-illness. She reports lethargy, fever and aching muscles, and that she's had a mildly sore throat and cough for a few days. During my examination I notice a distinctive almost perfect red triangle at the tip of her tongue. As an allopath I diagnose the flu, considering the appearance of the tip of her tongue to be an irrelevant detail (an "illegitimate" symptom). As a homeopath, I diagnose an acute case of *Rhus toxidendron* flu, because the appearance of her tongue is a specific symptom for this patient, and not common in flu generally. In making this diagnosis, I've noted *all* of her symptoms: common and uncommon, legitimate and illegitimate. In homeopathy, the little details or peculiarities often indicate the simillimum – the remedy that most similarly matches the symptoms for the individual. Such symptoms are commonly referred to as *strange, rare, or peculiar* symptoms (or SRPs). A red triangle at the tip of the tongue is known as a SRP for *Rhus tox.*

Traditional Chinese medicine (TCM), including acupuncture, also developed from the empirical method. In TCM, treatment is based on patterns of disharmony (or disruption of *chi* – loosely translatable as life force) expressed as symptoms; practitioners use all of their senses to directly observe these symptoms, and thereby gather the patterns. The pattern diagnosed needs to account for *all* the patient's symptoms. The equivalent of *chi* in homeopathy is the *vital force*. TCM, like homeopathy, is "based on an integrated coherent doctrine for its therapeutic practice", in Coulter's words, and is not appropriately assessed by a RCT.

Summary: rational vs empirical

Rationalist diagnosis makes use of a pre-existing theory. The physician's task is to interpret both the patient's symptoms and his own understanding of how medicines operate in the body, then attempt to correlate these two bodies of information with respect to the particular patient in front of him, making the process of diagnosis and treatment more an art than a science; it depends on the physician's judgement.

In contrast, in the empirical method, there is a direct methodological relationship between these two bodies of knowledge – the symptoms and the medicine (as in the Law of Similars). This means that research into therapies using the empirical method are not easily studied by research tools designed by and for those using the rationalist method. The RCT as a research tool for the rationalist method serves the purpose very well, but the same tool cannot be applied to homeopathy, due to the principle of individualisation that is characteristic of empirical medicine.

Yet homeopathy as an empirical method of medicine has somehow stood the test of time, even though it does not conform to the rationalist philosophy. In the following chapter we explore further how homeopathy may exert its effect in clinical practice.

CHAPTER FOUR

The Vital Force

Hahnemann's aphorisms

The sixth edition of Samuel Hahnemann's *Organon of Medicine* explains the principles of homeopathy as Hahnemann saw them, developed from his own observations during practical experience. His writing indicates a deep awareness of the interconnection of spirit, mind, and body in terms of health and disease. On reading the long introduction to the book, where Hahnemann proclaims the "evils" of allopathic medicine, it's not difficult to see how his perspective upset many of his allopathic medical colleagues. In this introduction, Hahnemann described those who applied both orthodox and homeopathic methods as "mongrels". I would be one such mongrel – but I truly believe that we now have the opportunity to move beyond a limited view of one or the other way of thinking, and recognise that homeopathy carries the potential for deeper healing, and rightfully belongs alongside orthodox medicine.

The *Organon* sets out a list of 291 *aphorisms*, or statements of the principles of homeopathy. Hahnemann's wholistic view of health and disease is demonstrated in aphorism 6: ". . . the changes in the health of the body and of the mind (morbid phenomena, accidents, symptoms) which can be perceived . . . represent the disease in its whole extent . . ."

He refers to "the affection of the vital force" as both the origin of disease and the place where restoration of health must occur in aphorism 7:

. . . the symptoms alone by which the disease demands and points to the remedy suited to relieve it – and moreover, the totality of these its symptoms, of this outwardly reflected picture of the internal essence of the disease, that is of the affection of the vital force, must be the principal or sole means whereby the disease can make known what remedy it requires . . . the only thing the physician has to take note of in every case of disease and to remove by means of his art in order that the disease shall be cured and transformed into health.

In aphorism 12, Hahnemann emphasises that a disease or derangement in the vital force is made known by an expression of symptoms revealing the whole disease, concluding that improvement in symptoms under treatment indicates a person's recovery:

It is the morbidly affected vital energy alone that produces diseases . . . they reveal the whole disease; also, the disappearance under treatment of all the morbid phenomena . . . implies the restoration of the integrity of the vital force and therefore the recovered health of the whole organism.

Most importantly, in aphorism 215, Hahnemann states there is no separation between diseases of the body (corporeal) and of the mind and emotions, as both are derangements of the same vital force: "Almost all the so-called mental and emotional diseases are nothing more than corporeal diseases . . ."

The vital force

One of the defining aspects of orthodox medicine is *dualism*, where mind and body are treated as separate parts of a person, as in a complex machine, while the life force is ignored. In all my years of medical training, I don't recall any reference to life force, or even what it means to be alive. The focus was on diagnosing and treating diseases. Near the end of training we received instruction on how to accurately, carefully, and medico-legally determine death, as defined by a *lack of vital signs*. Although a variety of bodily measurements might be included in this determination, in practice this refers to the absence of a heartbeat and the presence of fixed dilated pupils.

Many years ago, during my house officer years, a certain event occurred that comes to mind as I ponder the true meaning of vital force: paramount in homeopathy, yet somehow overlooked by orthodox medicine.

I was part of the on-call team in the hospital that day. My pager beeped an emergency signal indicating a patient in cardiac arrest on one of the wards. I didn't know the gentleman involved. He had no pulse and wasn't breathing, so we began CPR. I was in charge of his airway and breathing. I thought I must be doing a good job, as he quickly regained consciousness. He attempted to move and speak and the electrocardiograph displayed a reassuring signal of sinus rhythm, but there was still no pulse. When the anaesthetist arrived she took over the airway, and soon there wasn't anything for me to do but observe. At one point the patient sat up with wide staring eyes, attempting to speak. He looked shocked and anxious. I felt confused, as I knew the situation, called "pulseless electrical activity", was incompatible with life. His heart had stopped beating, and oxygen was only circulating in his blood because of external chest compression. Yet he appeared alive; animated with a vital force. Sadly, because the situation did not improve, and no reversible cause could be found, the other doctors ceased CPR and promptly departed, leaving two nurses and myself in the room. At this stage all we could do was hold the patient's hand for comfort and speak reassurances as the vital force left his body. It felt as if something important had been missed out in my training; all the technical instruction I had received hadn't prepared me for a situation like this.

Looking back now, I can see from a homeopathic perspective that this person was in an *Aconite* state. The homeopathic remedy *Aconite* is the simillimum for an acute case such as this, when sudden trauma on all levels leaves a person in shock and fear, with a sense of impending doom or imminent death. The patient might still be able to express this verbally, and physically they may look pale or flushed. They may have an anxious appearance, have difficulty breathing, and have a rapid bounding pulse, or later, a slowing feeble pulse. Administered as a spray into the mouth like the commonly used orthodox medicine for angina, I could argue a place for *Aconite* among conventional emergency equipment, in the hope that it might if possible maintain a person's vital force – or at least ease the process of passing.

There is now a growing field of mind–body medicine that conceptually integrates the illness experience of mind, body and spirit into a unified whole, to facilitate healing. Physician and psychotherapist Brian Broom shares stories of his clinical involvement with physical diseases that express patients' subjective experiences and life stories in *Meaning-Full Disease: How personal experience and meanings cause and maintain physical illness* (2007). He writes, "I believe we must consider the possibility that the (subject-) body has a fundamental vitality, spirit, and energy which can under certain circumstances be stifled or dysfunctional"(Broom, 2007, p. 155). His conclusion closely resembles Hahnemann's statement in aphorism 7, reproduced above.

Cellular biologist Bruce Lipton points out the relevance of modern physics to our biology in his book *The Biology of Belief* (2008). He cites Einstein's statement that E = mc^, meaning energy (E) = matter/mass (m) multiplied by the speed of light squared (c^), and goes on to suggest: "The Universe is one indivisible, dynamic whole in which energy and matter are so deeply entangled it is impossible to consider them as independent elements" (Lipton, 2008, p. 71).

Lipton explains how the discovery by quantum physics that atoms are constantly spinning and vibrating energy, each atom having a unique energy vibration or "signature", means that material structures in the universe, including ourselves, also radiate a unique electromagnetic energy signature.

This makes sense to a homeopath. In taking a case we listen carefully and observe all the symptoms of the patient, including mental, emotional, and physical symptoms, to obtain a complete signature of the illness, known as "the totality of symptoms". This signature information is specific and peculiar to the unique individual, and indicates the simillimum, or remedy providing the most similar match, needed as treatment. We already know that to have a healing effect homeopathy must interact with a person on an energetic level, due to ultra-dilution (see Chapter 3). It seems likely that, when the simillimum meets "the totality of symptoms" or signature energy of the individual, the similarity or resonance between them creates a change in the individual at a quantum-energy level.

The homeopathic definition of the vital force can be likened to *chi* in Traditional Chinese medicine or *prana* in Indian medicine, and encompasses what has been described as the human energy field (Brennan, 1988). I think that in reality our own energy fields are not truly separate from the universal energy field.

In homeopathy, disturbances in the vital force, expressed by symptoms, usually refer to an individual. An important exception involves the treatment of babies and children, who may express symptoms relating directly to a significant other: usually the mother, or another close family member. This isn't surprising considering the dynamic process of human reproduction and the progressive developmental stages of childhood. Homeopathic consultations for babies and children reflect this reality, encompassing information about the family, conception, pregnancy, labour, delivery, and beyond.

Sometimes a homeopath gives more than one person in a family the same remedy, or different remedies that have a certain relationship. If we think of symptoms or diseases as *information* indicating a disorder of the vital force, it makes sense that this information may be expressed by different members of a family unit. For the homeopath, eliciting information about several members of one family, or several generations, often provides greater insight to inform accurate remedy selection. Homeopaths who work with animals sometimes see a similar process occurring with people and their pets. Work with animals by biologist Rupert Sheldrake provides evidence to support such phenomena (Sheldrake, 2011).

The energy field in all of us

Barbara Ann Brennan's 1988 book *Hands of Light* describes the human energy field in detail. Although many of us are likely to have the innate ability to sense such things, we may lose that sensitivity as we grow up and realise that others don't typically share our experiences. I've encountered adults who report having seen colours around people as children, but have almost forgotten about it, and seem to have lost the ability.

Brennan explains that everyone has an energy field or aura surrounding and interpenetrating their physical body. Highly qualified, Brennan came to work in healing from a prior career as a research scientist for NASA; she has a masters degree in atmospheric physics. Brennan presents a simple exercise to start seeing auras (outlined below). I followed these instructions, and after initial success looking at the energy field surrounding a house plant, I soon discovered I could see my own energy field. Discovering this phenomenon for myself, with my own eyes, helped me understand where and how homeopathy might work. I introduced the technique to members of my GP peer group. After a short practice, in spite of initial nervousness and scepticism, they found they too could observe their own auras. By remaining relaxed and open-minded, readers can take the first step, and appreciate this intriguing phenomenon.

Exercise for seeing auras

A plain white wall provides an ideal background. It's best to start in a room where the light is slightly dim, with either natural light or a low level of light from behind, as looking into bright light makes it difficult for your eyes to diverge (move out of focus).

Hold both arms out in front of you at eye level with the fingertips facing each other, just a few centimetres apart. Look at the space between your hands, and allow your eyes to relax while maintaining the gaze. Don't try to focus on any one spot. Take your time.

Soon you will observe something in the space between your hands and around your fingers. Try slowly moving your fingers closer together to see what happens. Now try slowly moving them further apart. (Brennan, 1988, p. 42.)

Auras are not produced by a retinal after-image; they look and behave differently, as you will hopefully discover if you persist with the exercise above. They have an elastic mobile quality, and can vary in depth, brightness and colour depending on the viewer's perception, or with changes occurring in the person being viewed. It's worth practising a bit. If you do, your awareness may expand to include noticing auras around other people. Now that I've seen how the aura behaves, I can only assume it to be the manifestation of an energy field, and all my own observations so far seem to confirm this assumption.

After a little practice, I soon started noticing pale luminescent, mostly blue or green energy fields around other people; particularly at work while I was listening to a patient with my eyes relaxed, not focusing on a particular point. Seeing a person's aura involves looking beyond that person, or using your peripheral vision by looking at a part of them, while noticing what you see nearby at the periphery. The technique is much the same as that required to use the 3D *Magic Eye* books – you need to allow your eyes to diverge a little.

Because we see energy fields or auras using our peripheral vision, our ability to see colour and shape while doing so is lessened, as the parts of the retina used for peripheral vision have relatively fewer rod cells. The cone cells, concentrated at the fovea in the centre of the retina, can best detect colour and shape. To illustrate this: in dim lighting it can be difficult to see detail and colour if you look directly at an object, but if you use your peripheral vision, you will notice the object comes into better "focus". Having "opened my eyes" to this process, I now observe pale luminescent blue auras on the ceiling at home around recessed light fittings in dim light – presumably due to the electromagnetic fields they emit.

When I lent my copy of Brennan's book to a curious work colleague, the result was impressive. One day she burst into my room to report that "an unbelievable experience!" had just occurred during a consultation. She had been listening empathically while a patient related a very difficult problem that seemed unsolvable; she too was wondering what the solution might be, and asking herself what she could do to help. Suddenly she observed the periphery of the patient's body light up with a strong lime green-coloured aura. I had a similar experience several months later during an exercise at a training course: I saw a glowing lime green colour flickering around the edges of my own body. This also came as quite a surprise!

Electromagnetic fields are generally considered to be outside normal human visual perception: we typically only see light from 390 to 700 nanometre (nm) wavelength. However, these fields can be photographed with special equipment, as ultraviolet light is electromagnetic radiation with a shorter wavelength of 10 to 400 nm. People with aphakia (absence of the optical lens), which makes them long-sighted and unable to focus, can see ultraviolet light in a shorter than normal range of 300 to 400 nm. This creates a divergent gaze, engaging more of the peripheral retina, and provides a form of vision that is similar to that required to see auras.

Interconnecting energy

In *The Field* (2001), journalist Lynne McTaggart explores the evidence for a life force organising and interconnecting the energy fields of individuals and the world in which we live. She presents a broad view of the relevant science in an interesting and readable format. The book explores many fields of research, including a phenomenon known as photo-repair. This refers to the body's natural ability to repair cellular damage caused by ultraviolet light that occurs most efficiently at 380 nm, just outside the range of the normal visible spectrum of light. Biophysicist Fritz-Albert Popp performed research demonstrating that living organisms release "biophotons" or light energy; DNA is the most potent source of these photons. In research using a machine designed to measure this very low-intensity light, Popp discovered that certain insects, fish, and plants were both absorbing light and exchanging or sharing it, in a process he referred to as "photon sucking". This may explain the complex communicating systems at work within our bodies, because energy is a more efficient way of transferring information than chemicals. Popp suggests that homeopathic medicines may exert their action in the same way, behaving as a "resonance absorber", allowing the body to return to normal.

Science hasn't yet explained how living things, including human beings, transform from the division of a single cell into our three-dimensional form, but interesting theories have been presented. Biologist Harold Burr measured electrical fields surrounding living things. His experiments with salamanders (small lizards), capable of regenerating body parts that had been removed or lost, discovered an energy field shaped like an adult salamander within an unfertilised egg. The energy field appeared to behave like a map or blueprint, directing biological processes (Burr, 1972, as cited in McTaggart, 2003, p. 61).

Sheldrake put forward the concept of "morphogenic fields" to explain the apparent self-organisation that occurs throughout all biological systems. He uses the term "morphic resonance" to describe "the influence of like upon like through space and time" (Sheldrake, 1987, as cited in McTaggart, 2003, p. 60).

Such fields of resonance would help explain the complex communicating systems we observe in nature, both within living organisms and among them, extending even to the largest ecosystems, including the world in which we live.

Sheldrake's work is consistent with the key principle of homeopathy, which is quite simply, in Sheldrake's own words, "the influence of like upon like through space and time". I believe we can gain better understanding of how far this influence might extend by exploring our wider interconnections.

CHAPTER FIVE

Synchronicity: Connection Beyond Time and Space

Newtonian mechanics

Homeopathy is a valid empirical form of medicine, not *yet* fully explained. This is not surprising given how much of our own biology, and that of the natural world in which we live, remains a mystery.

Traditional linear models of information flow based on cause and effect, known as Newtonian mechanics, are too simplistic. In *Spontaneous Evolution* (2009) Lipton and Bhaerman summarise Sir Isaac Newton's science of mechanics: "Newton's science was based upon two absolutes: absolute space and absolute time. In a quantifiable Universe, as he defined it, objects move through these absolutes because of gravity" (Lipton and Bhaerman, 2009, p. 96).

Spontaneous Evolution goes on to elaborate on the three main tenets of Newtonian mechanics shaping scientific study: materialism ("All that matters is matter"), reductionism ("To understand something, take it apart and study its pieces"), and determinism ("We can predict and control the outcome of natural processes") (Lipton and Bhaerman, 2009, p. 96).

Consciousness shared

To fully grasp how our bodies work, we need to understand the nature of matter itself, and to explore our limited perceptions of the reality in which we live, including our subjectivity as observers. The laws of quantum physics have provided us with thought-provoking insights about how we relate to each other and absolutely everything in our environment. Under observation, subatomic matter, including that which makes up our own bodies, can be defined as a solid particle at a fixed location, yet when its momentum is measured it becomes a wave, in an effect known historically as the Heisenberg uncertainty principle. Such matter can therefore be defined in terms of "wave particles". Physician, Deepak Chopra, explains how significant we are as observers interacting with our environment, because *our consciousness* collapses the wave into the particle: "Without consciousness acting as an observer and interpreter, everything would exist only as pure potential. That pure potential is the virtual domain . . . that potential is what allows us to make miracles" (Chopra, 2003, p. 51).

Consciousness is not contained exclusively within our brains or our bodies. Numerous experiments demonstrating what is commonly known as ESP (extra-sensory perception) challenge our normal understanding of space and time. The concept of living beings interacting through organising energy fields that guide or regulate group behaviour is not new, and has been applied to phenomena observed among animals. Think of how flocks of birds fly in exact formation on apparently familiar migratory pathways, and how huge shoals of fish move, turning in unison.

Sheldrake's hypothesis of "morphic resonance" acting within "morphogenic fields" (Sheldrake, 1987) makes use of the idea of an accumulated form of memory that transcends space and time to explain the self-organising abilities of living things, not only within themselves, but interconnecting with other beings and the environment. Genetic theory doesn't explain such abilities.

One example of interconnected self-organising is widely known as the "hundredth monkey principle". This refers to the observation, documented by Lyall Watson in 1979, that after a group of monkeys on one island had learned a new behaviour, other monkeys on different islands, having had no physical interaction with the original group, quickly developed the same new behaviour – presumably by some form of group consciousness or coherence.

Those who have practised meditation will be aware that we somehow exist beyond the physical boundaries of our skin. One day, after sending my two young children off unaccompanied on a plane trip to meet their father, I turned my phone onto silent and settled into a quiet meditation, not expecting to be disturbed. My eyes were closed when an internal picture formed in my mind: at first I noticed their father, then my two girls beside him, bending over something together in a huddle. Momentarily annoyed at what I perceived as an intrusion on my meditation time, I thought no more of it, until later when I checked my mobile phone. A text from my children had arrived during the meditation; they had sent it from their father's phone to report their safe arrival, along with an abundance of hugs and kisses! Not only had I received their text via the mobile network; somehow I had also received additional information – an image of the senders – via my raised state of consciousness during meditation.

Synchronicity

Psychiatrist and psychotherapist Carl Jung used the word *synchronicity* to describe cases of meaningful coincidence. He likened the concept to that of Chinese *Tao*, and explored it in *Synchronicity: An Acausal Connecting Principle* (1960). While acknowledging the well-accepted law of cause and effect, or causality, Jung raised the possibility that the connection of certain circumstances – coincidences – required another principle of explanation, being *acausal*, but nonetheless connected.

As Jung experienced such coincidences and collected the stories of others, he noted how often the phenomena of synchronicity were associated with *archetypes*: symbols used by our unconscious seeking expression through conscious experience. Jung thought these archetypal images revealed innate individual tendencies that shaped human behaviour. While profoundly personal, they somehow also remain consistent across different cultures and times, as revealed by their appearance in art, literature, and mythology. These patterns provide a universal language for the internal expression of our connection with external reality.

The concept of synchronicity also describes how the *inner* symbolic experience of an individual manifests through meaningful occurrences in the *outer* physical reality.

Jung told of a young woman he had been treating without much success; he attributed this to her "Cartesian rationalism". The woman described to Jung a dream she had had in which she was given a golden scarab beetle brooch: an expensive piece of jewellery. Jung was sitting facing her with his back to the window as he listened to the story. He heard a gentle tapping sound, and, turning, saw a large flying insect knocking from outside against the dark glass. He opened the window and caught the scarabeid beetle, and noted its close resemblance to a golden scarab as he presented it to the woman, who apparently then progressed in treatment with satisfactory results. The scarab is known historically as a symbol of rebirth; an ancient Egyptian legend tells of the dead sun god changing himself into Chepri, the scarab, before being carried into the morning sky on a barge.

Surprisingly, synchronous events occurred for me on the exact day I researched and wrote the section above, at which point I had not previously heard of the sun-god legend. At work on this particular Monday, I happened to spend some time clearing a pile of papers that had lain on the floor beside my desk for around two years. I had been sharing my consulting room with a colleague for several months at that point, and I decided the clutter had to go. The only item I did not discard was a large envelope containing handwritten notes referring to two articles in a journal, also enclosed. I vaguely recalled a patient lending it to me after we had been discussing Paracelsus and the origins of homeopathic philosophy. The same evening, after writing about Jung's case, I decided to stop for the night, put my feet up and take a look at the journal for the first time. I was amazed to open it to a striking full-page colour photo of "The Scarab of Chepri" from the tomb of Tutankhamun, dating from 1323BC, depicting a symbol of the human being who bears the spiritual sun. A short while later, rising from my reading session, I wasn't as pleased to encounter a large cockroach on the wall right beside me!

Jung was interested in both alchemy and astrology, and how the inner experience of the individual related to the wider external reality of the cosmos. He sought to understand the interdependence of the individual and the collective. Late in 1913, he experienced a dream in which he saw a terrible flood covering all the northern and low-lying lands from England to Russia with waves and rubble, bringing death to thousands of people. The dream recurred two weeks later, yet more violently. Jung realised later, with the onset of war in July 1914, that his dream had related to a world event, rather than to his personal psychology.

I suspect this phenomenon is quite common, but one we don't talk about often, perhaps because the events they relate to are shocking, tragic or very personal for other people, and we don't see any direct link between those events and ourselves. The personal example I give here was not something I felt like sharing in the immediate aftermath of a local disaster.

Like most people I don't remember my dreams for long, unless they have particular significance, as occurred on Saturday 4 September 2010. I woke quite late in my home in Tauranga, and soon after learned of the advent of the first Canterbury earthquake, which had occurred at 4.35am. That morning, just after 3am, I had awoken from a dream in which the ground was moving beneath me and the building I was in. I felt and watched large waves move through the ground I was standing on. I heard no sounds, and felt no fear or threat. I was going in and out of houses, frustrated, as I tried without success to find one that wasn't moving. The houses were old buildings, reminding me, even at the time, of a familiar painting of an old schoolhouse in Christchurch. This is an example of synchronicity: no one would argue any causal link between the two events, my dream and the Canterbury earthquake.

It seems that where synchronicity occurs – that is, where events are linked yet acausal – our normal perception of time as linear is challenged. My dream occurred about an hour before the event it was connected with. Similarly, Jung's dream occurred months before war began. When we explore this concept, we start to realise the usual parameters of time and space are not a given. Many experiments have been carried out demonstrating the transfer of information by telepathy or "remote viewing" in a situation in which no direct contact was possible, due to differences in location and time. Sheldrake explores such "sixth sense" phenomena in *Dogs That Know When Their Owners Are Coming Home* (2011) and *The Sense of Being Stared At* (2003). If these titles make you feel uncomfortable, ask yourself why. Life is full of things we don't *yet* understand. Science hasn't *yet* explained so much about our world, but this doesn't mean we can ignore or discount it.

Over the years I've heard a number of patient stories regarding health problems involving synchronicity. One gentleman was confined to a wheelchair, the result of a neurological condition. He calmly explained to me how he had planned the wide double doorways in his home so they could accommodate a wheelchair years before he developed any symptoms. When the patient was young, his mother suffered from an unrelated condition threatening her ability to walk, but she recovered fully. Another woman has a daughter who was born with a genetic disorder for which there had been no family risk factors. She described being struck with an overwhelming feeling of concern late in the pregnancy, and when she had read about the particular disorder in a book: she had just *known* that her child would have the condition. At the same time she read about several other conditions, but these did not concern her. The feeling was confirmed a few weeks later, at the birth of her daughter.

The totality of symptoms

There are times and situations in which we "tune in" to certain information in an unrestricted way. This intuition or inner knowing is of supreme importance for healing. Personal meaning, revealed as patients tell their story, forms the basis of homeopathic case taking. The totality of symptoms on all levels, including that of the mind, reveals the simillimum homeopathic substance indicated as the remedy. The patient's story doesn't need to sound logical, demonstrate causality, or even make sense to the practitioner; it simply is.

In the mind–body split of orthodox medicine, mental factors are considered to be a cause of physical symptoms, described as *somatisation*. Similarly the word *psychosomatic* describes how psychological distress creates physical symptoms, but implies that these are simply "in the mind". The reverse holds true; the mind-body split recognises mental and emotional *effects* of physical illness, but still by a linear cause and effect model. In fact, the dynamics of human illness are much more complex: all the symptoms experienced form a unity (or totality), in a process best described as multifaceted.

Dr Brian Broom explores the subjective meaning of illness in *Somatic Illness and the Patient's Other Story: A practical integrative mind/body approach to disease for doctors and psychotherapists* (1997). Broom uses the prism as a metaphor to explain the illness experience to patients, demonstrating how we are multifaceted or multidimensional while still in the form of a unified whole. Broom points out that doctors have a valuable base of knowledge and expertise of their own; however, he says that doctors can only discover the *meaning* of a patient's illness through working with that individual.

I was fortunate to attend one of Brian Broom's workshops many years ago after beginning my study of homeopathy, and was enthused by the similarity of the homeopathic and Broom's integrative approaches to illness. Dr Broom gave a personal account of his own illness experience concerning an unusual skin lesion on his arm. He told us that he had known intuitively that this had particular meaning. In the event, the lesion completely resolved during psychotherapy; this profound experience was what spurred Broom on to further work in mind–body medicine, utilising the psychotherapeutic process as treatment.

In my experience, counselling or psychotherapy are often beneficial during homeopathic treatment, in which conscious awareness tends to develop around issues previously unconscious or suppressed. Counselling and psychotherapy are ways to safely explore and resolve these issues. My experience has also been that homeopathic treatment can help patients become conscious of (and facilitate resolution of) issues that have not been resolved in psychotherapy (see the second case discussed in Chapter 9), so the two are complementary therapies.

Patients' ability to reveal the remedy they need

Homeopathic doctor Edward Whitmont explores the relationship between a person's subjective experience of disease and the homeopathic remedy in *Psyche and Substance* (1986). Whitmont also analyses the archetypal forms of various remedies in the context of Jungian psychology. While there are other methodologies in homeopathic case analysis, most homeopaths agree that the subjective sensations revealed through a patient's symptoms often indicate the specific remedy that patient needs.

Linda Johnston, MD and homeopath, has published many detailed cases of patients expressing their simillimum so clearly through their *sensations* (physical, mental, and emotional) that they spontaneously and eloquently reveal the substance they need for healing (Vermeulen & Johnston, 2011). So that the practitioner can follow the patient's *sensation* or *feeling*, it's important for the patient to feel relaxed and safe; this facilitates the free flow of information and associations, allowing what may be unconscious to be revealed. A skilled and experienced homeopath may then observe, listen, and guide the patient only to the extent necessary to find the indicated remedy.

One of Johnston's case examples illustrates how strongly one female patient identified with a substance that turned out to be the appropriate remedy: *Taraxicum* or dandelion. In reply to the homeopath's request to describe her intense anger a little more, the patient said:

> It is a dandelion! (She looks triumphant as if it all makes complete sense to her). The wind comes unexpectedly and blows away the soft flower head and all that is left is the stripped flower stalk. It was pretty and soft, now it is hard and ugly. That is me. As a child my mother would be the

unexpected wild storm and blow away my softness . . . (Vermeulen & Johnson, 2011, Vol. 1, p. 769).

The genus epidemicus and miasms

Just as an individual person may experience symptoms indicating resonance with a substance or remedy at a particular time, families and groups of people can experience similar symptoms that collectively indicate such resonance. The homeopathic term *genus epidemicus* refers to a single remedy that a homeopath finds to be appropriate for multiple sufferers of a particular epidemic. It may be applied when patients experience common symptoms of acute infectious diseases. The symptomatology of each epidemic is distinctive for that epidemic; no two epidemics are alike in this respect. Hahnemann referred to treatment during epidemics in his *Organon of Medicine* (aphorisms 100 to 102). He considered that carefully observant homeopaths could select an appropriate remedy or remedies early on, providing them with the potential to treat new cases as they arose. Whether such remedies are effective as *prophylaxis* (that is, a treatment given to *prevent* disease) against the same disease is more controversial; the idea needs to be considered in the light of a *collective* experience of disease.

In the early days of homeopathy, there was not yet knowledge about a clear connection between specific contagious diseases and their causative micro-organisms. The main theory of causation at the time was "miasma", which literally meant "bad air"; it's not surprising that Hahnemann used this same word to explain the origins of chronic diseases, which were more difficult to treat. He postulated a hereditary aspect to these diseases, and he classified three "miasms" according to his observations of the diseases (syphilis, gonorrhoea, and scabies) with which they were associated even though genetics had not yet been discovered.

The concept of miasms is still important in homeopathy today as a way of understanding and treating what might be described as *predisposing patterns of disease expression*, which have their origins in heredity, indicated by family history, and in response to the environment. If such predisposing patterns can be successfully treated with homeopathy, there is the potential to alter disease expression in future generations. Lipton (2008) suggests that genes do not equate to destiny, because environmental signals control the activity of genes. Chromosomal DNA is passed on, but environmental influences can change the expression of genes by changing the protein sleeve coating DNA, which determines what genes are able to be read. This has been demonstrated by researchers in the field of "epigenetics" (which means "control above genetics").

Conclusion

To put it simply, we live in a much more complex world than the orthodox bio-medical model of illness would suggest. Our current level of scientific knowledge does not define this world. In spite of my training and work within those same limitations, over the years life has pushed me into experiences that took me beyond those confines, leading me to question them. Cracks in the walls surrounding the medical system are perhaps most easily visible from the other side. Over the years, such experiences "outside" the borders have occurred at points at which my family, myself, and my colleagues have entered the system as patients, and discovered a very different viewpoint.

CHAPTER SIX

The Little Girl and the Dragon

This is the true story of a sick little girl and her magic dragon.
I have chosen it to illustrate how individuals interconnect and
share information with the wider field of consciousness
through meaningful coincidences, in a process known as
synchronicity. This little girl's story reveals how the hidden
meaning of illness is often completely overlooked by orthodox
medical diagnosis and treatment.

A mystery illness

In September 2006, when our youngest daughter, Georgia,
was just six, she became unwell. She showed all the typical
symptoms of viral illness: fevers, nausea, lethargy, and loss of
appetite. However, she recovered after about two weeks, and
returned to school for the last term of the year.

During the summer holidays that followed, she returned
from a long car trip very tired. In the first week of school she
developed symptoms that were very similar to those that she'd
had with her illness four months prior – only this time she
didn't improve. She became increasingly unwell. When she
became jaundiced, she was admitted to hospital. At the
hospital she remained sick and feverish. Her blood tests
showed elevated liver enzymes and a low white cell count, and
she wasn't getting better.

Deeply concerned, I phoned our homeopath for advice. I
explained all Georgia's symptoms, including those she'd had
during the recent illness, and the homeopath asked about her
mental and emotional symptoms. Georgia had been irritable
and had expressed a volatile temper for a few weeks, I told

her; it was mostly directed at me. Her father and I had separated eighteen months earlier, and she seemed to be coping fine, but lately there had been angry outbursts. She hadn't been happy about leaving "the big house", with her much loved sandpit, when we'd sold the property after the separation. The homeopath responded by prescribing *Magnesium mur* (chloride salt of magnesium) 200c. She explained that she had chosen *Magnesium mur* for the angry child (*Mur*) of separating parents (*Mag*); she considered that Georgia's anger toward her mother had shown as jaundice from inflammation of the liver (*Mur*). Under the circumstances this had made sense, so I went ahead and gave Georgia the remedy.

Within a day or two Georgia's temperature dropped, and her liver tests normalised. Although her white blood cell count remained very low, she was allowed home on the eighth day, with a diagnosis of viral illness as the cause of everything. We agreed to repeat the blood count later that week to check that her white cells were recovering.

Serial blood tests after that continued to indicate low white blood cell levels. Meanwhile, however, Georgia seemed well. She returned to her new class at school, and attended dance lessons again. A further week went by and then a few immature white cells, called blasts, were reported in her blood film. The doctors thought these were possibly a result of her bone marrow recovering from the effects of the virus. Two days later the doctors saw many blast cells in the blood film. This raised suspicion of leukaemia.

We arranged an urgent trip to Auckland for bone-marrow testing. However, it was now well over two weeks since Georgia had appeared to "recover", so I hoped it was all some terrible mistake.

Every parent's nightmare

At this time our homeopath prescribed *Aurum phos* (phosphorous salt of gold) 200c, for grief (*Aurum*) going to the blood or bones (*Phos*).

On the car journey to Auckland, Georgia recounted to me a dream she'd had the night before. Our whole family had been living happily in a house on top of a green hill surrounded by green land and other hills. An image of Teletubby land formed in my mind. I saw a glimpse of what my child naturally wanted: her family back together again, living happily ever after. Two days later, I could see that her illness had in a way achieved this for her. There we both were, her father and I, together at her bedside working through the practicalities of every parent's nightmare.

On day one in Auckland, the bone marrow result confirmed acute lymphoblastic leukaemia. The doctor informed me of the treatment plan and prognosis. There would be a month of intensive chemotherapy in Starship Children's Hospital aiming to achieve remission, followed by two years and two months of less intensive chemotherapy. We could return home after the first month, they told us, and thereafter take regular trips to Auckland and sometimes the local hospital.

The specialist we saw was confident Georgia's original presentation to the local hospital with fever, jaundice, and vomiting had been typical of acute leukaemic crisis, but could offer no explanation as to why she had improved and appeared to recover for so long. I hadn't mentioned the *Mag mur* to anyone at the time I'd given it to Georgia. Now I realised that this may have helped her recover, but had not resolved the underlying disease. Perhaps the remedy had been close but not an exact simillimum; or perhaps she needed more frequent doses because the illness was intense and progressing rapidly.

In acute leukaemia, white cell numbers rise exponentially, doubling every one or two days, as abnormal white blood cells pour into the bloodstream. For the best prognosis, Georgia needed immediate orthodox treatment.

A stand-off

The regime of chemotherapy proposed by the specialist had a long-term cure rate in the higher nineties; we had no difficulty agreeing to it. However, I was astounded to be told I couldn't treat my daughter with homeopathy alongside it! As a GP and homeopath, I knew that homeopathy was completely safe; there was no risk of interference or interaction with the chemotherapy. The problem was that the oncologist didn't know about homeopathy, and wasn't listening to me. It was a double blow for me to receive news confirming Georgia's diagnosis of leukaemia and also to hear that she couldn't have the additional treatment I considered so important, to treat her illness on all levels and help manage the inevitable side effects of chemotherapy.

I complained to a nurse on the ward, who kindly presented me with the hospital's "Alternative Therapies Policy", a small folder containing advice and a few articles dated 1990-something; there was no mention of homeopathy. It was now 2007, so I wasn't impressed. I was deprived of sleep, and my indignation rose swiftly. During the night I informed the duty nurse I wanted an opportunity to discuss homeopathy with another doctor in the morning. If it wasn't granted to me, I said, I would be protesting outside the front door of the hospital, and they could expect to see me on the TV news that night!

The next morning a large group of people on the ward round arrived in our room. The oncologist asked me if I'd "come to my senses" about my daughter's treatment.

In a phone conversation the evening before, my homeopath had quite reasonably suggested to me that I ignore the rules and give the remedy anyway, because we knew it was safe. However, I considered that there was a bigger principle at stake. Now, in front of a large group of witnesses, I carefully explained about the infinitesimal dose, and how a homeopathic remedy was chosen.

At last I was heard. The oncologist understood now that no material substance remained at a molecular level in the homeopathic remedy, and allowed me to administer the treatment. This discussion having taken place, the oncologist promptly turned and departed, and I watched in confusion as a line of people followed. Apparently, if the homeopathic remedy contained "nothing", there was no need to even record it on the drug chart. A social worker stayed behind to talk with me. There had been occasional cases where inappropriate substances had been given to patients during treatment, the social worker explained; this could be dangerous. I understood this, and understood why our doctor had been so concerned. Following this stand-off, we enjoyed a great relationship with the oncologist and all the staff involved in Georgia's treatment. We felt immensely reassured by their expertise, and remain very grateful for all their wonderful care.

Georgia received multiple treatments, given as tablets, infusions, and injections, along with transfusions, procedures, and anaesthetics. These were counted with a growing string of "bravery beads" presented by the nurses to acknowledge each medical intervention. She had regular courses of steroids, along with antibiotics and antiviral medications to help prevent infections during the times when this little patient was most vulnerable, and her immune system severely compromised. I gave her a number of homeopathic remedies to help manage side effects. The plant remedies I gave were *Aconite*, *Arnica*, *Ignatia*, *Nux vomica*, and *Pulsatilla*. The mineral remedies I gave were *Arsenicum album*, *Borax*, *Mercurius solubis*, and *Radium bromatum*. I also gave honey bee poison: *Apis*.

Georgia's strong-willed nature was both a hindrance and a blessing to her as she tried to gain control of a frightening situation. At the beginning she refused to swallow medicines, so the nurses used nasogastric tubes to administer treatment directly to her stomach. She frequently vomited these back up. Eventually she took on the challenge, and learnt to swallow a handful of tablets in one gulp. She missed a lot of school, and spent days at home playing alone when her white cell count was dangerously low so she was not allowed out, or suffering from the side effects of chemotherapy.

Draggy is lost

One memorable day during this time, Georgia was celebrating her soft toy Draggy's first birthday. It had been twelve months since she had won this small colourful toy dragon at a fair.

Draggy is striking in appearance, made from bright purple and yellow velvet, with a crop of red hair, matching red claws, and a cheeky grin revealing his single large tooth. He measures only 10 cm tall because his legs are too floppy to take his weight. He sits in front of me now, grinning mischievously as I write.

We had a morning appointment at the local hospital for intramuscular chemotherapy. Georgia knew it would hurt, so she was bringing Draggy along too, and her favourite teddy. Following the treatment I suggested we might have morning tea out as a treat. But Georgia was more interested in getting to the library that day than anything else. Leaving the car outside the library, I saw her stuff Draggy into her pocket, and warned her, "Don't bring Draggy; you might lose him!" But Georgia insisted, because it was Draggy's birthday. She said that, to celebrate, they were looking for a favourite library book with a dragon-shaped birthday cake on the cover. So off we went.

Inside the library a short time later, Georgia called out to me in alarm: "Mum! Draggy's gone! I lost him!" Distressed and crying, she led the librarian and me to the spot where she had been standing looking at books when Draggy disappeared out of her pocket. The three of us looked around the bookshelves as well as in the children's area, but we couldn't find him anywhere. I got down with my head on the floor to double check. The shelves were elevated on legs, leaving space beneath, so I could scan the entire room this way. It was terribly upsetting, but eventually we had to leave and just hope the staff would find him – or perhaps he would be handed in.

I drove home feeling somehow responsible for what had happened. I had told Georgia not to bring Draggy along because he might get lost, and the negative situation I had envisaged had indeed eventuated. A memory surfaced in my mind. The night before, I had begun reading a book called *The Lightworker's Way*, by Doreen Virtue (1997). In the first chapter Virtue describes a crisis episode from a day in her own childhood, when she had left her favourite little red purse behind while out playing. Her mother had told her, "Nothing is lost in the eyes of God"; in the morning, she had woken to find the purse right beside her bed.

I knew the power of belief, and I didn't want our sick child stressing, particularly now when we were working toward her recovery. I reassured Georgia that Draggy couldn't possibly be gone, because dragons don't just disappear – he must've run away to be cheeky, or been abducted by another child visiting the library. As I spoke, trying to convince myself too, Georgia joined in with my guessing game; we discussed all the possible mischief Draggy might be getting up to. Of course, we said, he would eventually get bored and come home – or perhaps he'd be so naughty that the person who stole him or found him would want to bring him back.

It was a difficult time. In spite of our phoning the library and dropping in several times to take another look, Draggy remained lost. We tried to keep our hopes and intentions focused on his safe return.

The magic dragon

About six weeks later, it was time to return to hospital for another chemotherapy injection. After the treatment, Georgia asked to go to the library again. She wouldn't accept my suggestion that we perhaps go to the other library in town today. When we walked in, I was surprised by a large cardboard cut-out picture on the library desk, depicting a large dragon smiling down at a small girl! He was advertising Book Week. I made another hopeful enquiry after the missing soft toy, but the librarian told me there was no sign of him.

My discussion with the librarian was interrupted by Georgia calling from across the library, "Mum, Mum, It's Draggy! He came back!" She stood smiling triumphantly, holding up the familiar cheeky toy. I hurried over, followed by two librarians, both shaking their heads in astonishment and muttering words like "weird" and "creepy". Georgia had found Draggy lying on the carpet in the exact same spot where he had disappeared six weeks earlier.

There was no three-dimensional, "rational" explanation for what had occurred. My sick little eight-year-old was not capable of staging such a hoax. How had Draggy disappeared in the first place, and where had he been? The most likely scenario, of Draggy sitting quietly on the bookshelf somehow concealed, and then spontaneously falling onto the floor on the right day at the exact time his owner walked in (past a stand-up picture of a dragon and a little girl on the counter), was hard to believe. Perhaps he had been taken, then returned at *just the right time?*

It was obvious to all of us that something very special, defying any logical causal explanation, had occurred.

Dragons, like Puff in the well-known song, represent magic. Traditionally they're associated symbolically with the "hero" archetype of our ego – the hero fights to slay the dragon. In this case Draggy was the hero, magically returning to his owner after a six-week adventure, during which she maintained her faith in his safe return. This faith helped Georgia through a long process of treatment and recovery.

Here Draggy sits now grinning back at me, his plush colourful fabric a palpable reminder of the stuff of miracles.

CHAPTER SEVEN

One Man's Poison

Several years ago I experienced some unusual physical symptoms. They showed up for the first time during a procedure I had to treat troublesome varicose veins, then recurred later, revealing a series of synchronicities I couldn't ignore. The result was my inspiration to one day write a book to share my experiences with homeopathy.

Symptoms without a rational explanation

At my appointment to treat the varicose veins, as I lay prone on a treatment table having a tiny amount of local anaesthetic injected into my calf, I began to feel an odd sensation. I felt numbness and mild pins and needles creeping slowly up my leg. Just as it reached my thigh, I noticed the same sensation moving up the other leg. Automatically thinking bio-medically, I could not find a rational explanation for this experience. Soon both my legs felt completely numb and impossibly heavy, so I decided to speak up. The surgeon hesitated a few moments and then he laughed, reassuring me it wasn't possible for his injection to cause the symptoms I was experiencing. He admitted my comment had initially surprised him: recently, when he had been injecting local anaesthetic into a patient's wound for pain relief, he had unintentionally caused a femoral nerve block, leaving the unfortunate person unable to stand for several hours.

My legs continued to feel numb and heavy for a while, but the weakness wore off by the time I needed to stand and walk again, so I didn't think any more about it.

A visit to my colleague

A few months earlier, a medical colleague of mine had been diagnosed with a form of cancer, unfortunately incurable by orthodox medicine. She was now very unwell. One day, I went to visit her at her home, located at the top of a hill. While I was driving slowly up the steep winding road, I started to experience the same sensation of numbness and heaviness, at first in my feet and steadily creeping higher as I approached my destination. This time it seemed worse: my legs felt weak as I struggled out of the car and walked slowly to the door. I was baffled by the return of these symptoms. On entering the house, I noticed two red jackets already hanging on hooks. I removed my own jacket – also red – and hung it up beside them. The jackets belonged to the two doctors who lived in the house. They seemed to be a reminder of what I had in common with this couple; we all had an interest in complementary therapies and healing paradigms beyond the limitations of orthodox medicine.

During my visit I heard how hopeless and powerless this couple had felt when, after the diagnosis, they had heard that there was no treatment with any hope of cure, and when their ideas about pursuing other forms of healing had been discounted without support or acknowledgement. I wished I'd made contact earlier, but I hadn't wanted to interfere, and I didn't know whether homeopathy could alter my colleague's severely weakened state. In the current medical model, the state of knowledge is that particular conditions – including many forms and stages of cancer – are incurable, and that many complementary therapies are "unproven". As I discussed in Chapter 3, the orthodox medical yardstick, the randomised controlled trial, is not an appropriate tool for measuring empirical medicine such as homeopathy. We simply don't know, and therefore can't say, what effect individualised empirical therapies that integrate mind and body as a whole might have in any given situation.

The nocebo effect

Unfortunately the medical prognosis "incurable" can have a strong negative impact on patients. In the well-recognised placebo effect, positive expectations can result in an improvement in health. Conversely, in the *nocebo effect*, negative expectations can result in negative outcomes. The word nocebo means in Latin "I shall harm". In medical interactions, comments about diagnosis and prognosis can therefore have a positive or a negative effect. As doctors we need to choose our words carefully, because (whether we are aware of it or not ourselves) those words form part of both a "disease" and its "treatment".

It's well documented that our beliefs affect our biology in a tangible way. We may be conscious of these beliefs or we may not – and often our subconscious beliefs are much more powerful. Lipton (2008) points out that the conscious mind is the creative one; we might use it to try to apply positive thinking. In contrast, the much more powerful subconscious mind contains a huge amount of learned (programmed) beliefs and responses accumulated over entire lives; these can easily sabotage our best intentions. The teaching and programming a young doctor receives at medical school and as he or she enters the orthodox medical world beyond serve as an example of a powerful process of "indoctrination" into a particular belief system.

I returned home from the visit to my colleague feeling hopeless and powerless. I had perceived that she was in the end stage of a difficult illness. She was now confined to bed, and had been too weak to even talk much. She had tried some complementary therapies, but without any recognition from the practitioners of orthodox medicine she'd been seeing.

I wanted to recommend a homeopathic remedy, but was worried that it might be too little too late. I wondered how to make a remedy choice from the limited information I had of my colleague's personal story. With no other option, I simply "asked" for help. An answer came quickly: the word *Conium* popped into my head. It was the name of a remedy I knew but hadn't prescribed before, so I looked it up. Poison hemlock is the common name for *Conium maculatum*. As I read and was reminded of the effects of this poisonous plant, slowly ascending paralysis starting at the feet, I was surprised by their similarity to my own recent experiences. *Conium* is known also as a remedy for slowly progressive insidious cancers and tumours. It seemed like a reasonable choice for my colleague, and we agreed that she would start this homeopathic remedy the following week. However, given the advanced stage of her illness, her peaceful passing some days later was no surprise to me. I continued to ponder the significance of it all.

Exploring the synchronicity

Eventually I decided to take a dose of homeopathic *Conium* myself. I had experienced those symptoms first during the vein procedure and again when I was driving up the steep hill to visit my sick colleague; perhaps my own symptoms were revealing a simillimum remedy for me. One day, after finishing up at work, I popped a couple of pilules into my mouth and locked up my office. Once the sugar dissolves under your tongue it's easy to forget about taking a remedy. Often life just carries on – unless something unusual occurs, as it did this time. For the third time, my symptoms started again. Just as I was driving up the incline of the Harbour Bridge, I felt the now familiar tingling creeping numbness of my feet moving slowly higher. As I neared home the frustrating weakness made it difficult for me to use the foot pedals; at one point, a car behind me at an intersection tooted as I moved off very slowly. On reaching home I lifted my legs out of the car and moved carefully to lie on the bed. I reassured my family and myself that it was just a strange symptom which would soon wear off!

I knew there were two possible explanations for this third episode of similar symptoms. It's possible that I was "proving" the remedy *Conium*, just temporarily experiencing some of the symptoms associated with this homeopathic remedy. However, given that I had first felt the sensation during the vein procedure, and that once this third episode had resolved, after about ten minutes, the symptoms never returned, I believe this was the simillimum for my "acute" problem. My experience of such inexplicable symptoms, which could best be described as "iatrogenic" (caused by medical treatment) in the first instance – and the fact that the symptoms returned when they did – only seemed to make sense in the light of synchronicity.

I recalled noticing a book by Dan Millman, successful athlete and inspirational writer, on the coffee table during the visit to my colleagues' home. I had read one of his books, *Way of the Peaceful Warrior* (1985), many years ago, and by chance had read it again when my daughter was in hospital. Perhaps it was important. What was the name of that character? I racked my brain for the answer, knowing it was hidden there somewhere. At last it came: Socrates, of course! Suddenly I saw a connection between Socrates, the homeopathic remedy *Conium*, and my recurring symptoms of slowly ascending numbness with paralysis.

Plato (c.428–c.348BC) recorded the symptoms experienced by Socrates (460–399BC) after he was condemned to death by drinking poison hemlock; these contributed to the body of information used by homeopaths today, and included the symptoms I had been experiencing.

Seeking to understand the meaning of the synchronicity I was observing, I decided to learn more about the life and teachings of the famous philosopher himself.

Socrates' life and death

In my research, and in my discussion here, I have drawn on historian Bettany Hughes' beautifully detailed and candid biography of Socrates, *The Hemlock Cup: Socrates, Athens and the Search for the Good Life* (2010).

All we know about Socrates comes from the writings of others: Socrates himself didn't believe in writing things down, because he considered no debate was possible with the written word. Socrates lived in classical Greek Athens at a time described as the birth of democracy. He famously questioned the world around him, including the politics and values of the time. He pointed out that persuasive speeches in the new people-powered democracy didn't necessarily reveal *truth*.

Socrates rejected the pursuit of materialism and power. He wore a simple light robe, and went barefoot all year round. In spite of his philosophical questioning, he remained respectful of religious customs, and obeyed the city's laws. Some of his ideas were radical to his peers; particularly his notion that beauty and goodness were not necessarily associated with ideal physical attributes. In the Athens of the times, such attributes were popularly believed to be signs of inner beauty. Socrates' motivation was to examine and understand both himself and the human condition. It was Socrates who said "The unexamined life is not a life worth living for a human being" (Hughes, 2010, citing Plato's *Apology*, p. xvii).

Socrates' interest in what it meant to be human – to live and die – influenced many cultures through history, including Islamic tradition and the Western world. Since Socrates first formulated it, many have applied his "Socratic method", using question and counter-question and drawing from his simple, humble statement, "I know that I do not know".

Socrates' questioning of the status quo did not go unnoticed by those in power. He was charged and found guilty of disrespect for the city of Athens' gods, introducing new divinities, and corrupting the young. The verdict was decided by a majority of only 30 from 500 votes made in a democratic court. As a result, Socrates was famously and tragically sentenced to death. Hughes maintains that "He was the first person who really talked about human life; and he was also the first philosopher who was condemned to death and executed" (Hughes, 2010, p. 329, citing Diogenes Laertius, *The Lives and Opinions of Eminent Philosophers, Socrates, V*).

It is interesting – and remains somewhat of a mystery – that, at the moment before his death, Socrates spoke of a sacrifice to the god of healing. He said: "Crito, we owe a cock to Asclepius, make this offering to him and do not forget" (Hughes, 2010, p. 351, citing Plato, *Phaedo* Trans. Grube, 1997). Asclepius was a relatively new god at the time. Symbolic pictures of this deity – the familiar long staff wrapped with a snake – are still used today to represent medicine and healing. I have a photo of myself taken years ago standing in front of a statue of Asclepius at the National Museum of Athens. I still recall the excitement I felt coming face to face with this historical figure.

It seems Socrates made the ultimate sacrifice in giving up his own life to humanity. What is the relevance of this to homeopathy, health, and healing?

Becoming acquainted with our souls

I believe the answer lies in Socrates' clear interest in and pursuit of the meaning of human life and consciousness, including death. Concepts including what it means to be human, the way we experience the world, and our beliefs and values remain conspicuously absent from current orthodox medicine. However, all cultures use art, literature, music, and drama to celebrate meaning in human lives. The bio-medical model of orthodox medicine has developed as a doctrine devoid of the role of *meaning* in illness and disease, on the basis that this is somehow "scientific".

To question the assumptions of the scientific method makes many of us uncomfortable, because it has far-reaching implications. Inevitably, we are led to question the very reality in which we live. But understanding that the long-established medical model has a somewhat one-sided and limited view is essential to our ability to move beyond its rigid structure, and allow true healing to occur. It's not that the orthodox medical thinking is wrong. We know it works – but only as far as it goes. The scientific world does not explain, define, or limit the real world in which we live as individuals, and there is still much to learn from thinkers like Socrates, whose main concern was with the world *as lived*.

In his thinking in this regard, Broom explores Husserl's concept of *lebenswelt*, which translates to "life-world", and its relevance to health and disease:

> Quite simply, the life-world is a rich, multidimensional, experienced reality of which the scientific world is a part-representation, a reduction, or an abstraction. The life-world is of such a nature that it does have geometrical (and other) forms, such as volumes, surfaces, edges, and intersections, which therefore have measureable aspects. But the life-world is not fully comprehended in all its richness by science, because science is the methodology by which the physical forms of the life-world can be explored. (Broom, 2007, p. 101)

Socrates was most interested in what is *within* us: "He who orders us to know ourselves is bidding us to become acquainted with our soul" (Hughes, 2010, p. xx). He believed in dialogue; that open conversation is essential for the psyche, and works in a cathartic way. The Greek word used by Plato is "katharsis", meaning "releasing bad things". When Socrates talked about care of the soul, he suggested true happiness can only be achieved when we are at peace with ourselves. It is my belief that health and happiness are inextricably linked: our inner perspective has a huge impact on our health. How we perceive and integrate suffering in turn affects our quality of life and that of those around us.

The wise philosopher suggested it is "us", not "them", who can make things better. This idea refers to our innate ability to heal ourselves. It requires us to look inside ourselves for the *meaning* of our symptoms, and our suffering. Medical interventions bring with them the accumulation of vast amounts of knowledge and expertise, yet healing occurs within us. This wisdom opens up a whole new paradigm in medicine.

CHAPTER EIGHT

A New Paradigm in Medicine

"Sometimes the questions are complicated and the answers are simple"
~ Dr Seuss

My homeopath colleague recently asked me what progress I was making with the writing of this book. I told her that I was satisfied with drafts of the first seven chapters, some of Chapter 9 was completed, and I had a plan for concluding with Chapter 10, but that Chapter 8 was still holding me back. I said I felt pressured and tense, as if the task was too big and the words wouldn't flow. My efforts to find time and opportunities to write were often obstructed. She was quick to point out, "Of course number eight is the most difficult stage!" At this point everything started to make sense to me. The outer reality was reflecting my inner reality – or was my inner reality responding to the outer reality? One didn't really cause the other, they were just *similar.*

Stage eight

I had been taking a homeopathic remedy called *Samarium phosphoricum* for the difficult task (*Samarium*) of communicating (*Phos*) about homeopathy with non-homeopaths. I was having migraines that were increasing in intensity and duration the harder I tried to break through my sense of difficulty. I had left general practice two months earlier with the intention to finish this book and work more with homeopathy. Since then everything had felt difficult and I lacked energy – I had even been asking others if they noticed how heavy and thick the atmosphere was!

Figure 1: The periodic system of the elements

Periodic system of the elements

Homeopathy and the Elements (2002), reproduced by arrangement with Jan Scholten.

1	2	3	4	5	6	7	8	9
1 H Hydrogen								
3 Li Lithium	4 Be Berylium	5 B Boron						
11 Na Natrium	12 Mg Magnesium	13 Al Aluminium						
19 K Kalium	20 Ca Calcium	21 Sc Scandium	22 Ti Titanium	23 V Vanadium	24 Cr Chromium	25 Mn Manganum	26 Fe Ferrum	27 Co Cobaltum
37 Rb Rubidium	38 Sr Strontium	39 Y Yttrium	40 Zr Zirconium	41 Nb Niobium	42 Mo Molybdenum	43 Tc Technetium	44 Ru Ruthenium	45 Rh Rhodium
55 Cs Caesium	56 Ba Barium	57 La* Lanthanum	72 Hf Hafnium	73 Ta Tantalum	74 W Tungsten	75 Re Rhenium	76 Os Osmium	77 Ir Iridium
87 Fr Francium	88 Ra Radium	89 Ac** Actinium						
		57 La* Lanthanum	58 Ce Cerium	59 Pr Praseodymium	60 Nd Neodymium	61 Pm Promethium	62 Sm Samarium	63 Eu Europium
		89 Ac** Actinium	90 Th Thorium	91 Pa Protoactinium	92 U Uranium	93 Np Neptunium	94 Pu Plutonium	95 Am Americium

10	11	12	13	14	15	16	17	18
								2 He Helium
6 C Carbon					7 N Nitrogen	8 O Oxygen	9 F Fluor	10 N Neon
14 SI Silicium					15 P Phosphorus	16 S Sulphur	17 Cl Chlorum	18 A Argon
28 Ni Niccolum	29 Cu Cuprum	30 Zn Zincum	31 Ga Gallium	32 Ge Germanium	33 As Arsenicum	34 Se Selenium	35 Br Bromium	36 Kr Krypton
46 Pd Palladium	47 Ag Argentum	48 Cd Cadmium	49 In Indium	50 Sn Stannum	51 Sb Antimonium	52 Te Tellurium	53 I Iodium	54 Xe Xenon
78 Pt Platinum	79 Au Aurum	80 Hg Mercurius	81 Tl Thallium	82 Pb Plumbum	83 Bi Bismuth	84 Po Polonium	85 At Astatinum	86 Rn Radon
64 Gd Gadolinium	65 Tb Terbium	66 Dy Dysprosium	67 Ho Holmium	68 Er Erbium	69 Tm Thulium	70 Yb Ytterbium	71 Lu Lutetium	
96 Cm Curium	97 Bk Berkelium	98 Cf Californium	99 Es Einsteinium	100 Fm Fermium	101 Md Mendelevium	102 No Nobelium	103 Lw Lawrencium	

Homeopathic physician Jan Scholten introduced the concept of stages in the first edition of his book *Homeopathy and the Elements* in 1996. His work refers to the eighteen stages (groups) of elements that appear across the periodic table (Figure 1), from left to right. The periodic table is well known in chemistry. It lists all the chemical elements in order of increasing atomic number; within it, groups and rows reflect similar chemical properties of the known elements. There is space in the table for new elements yet to be discovered. The table provides us with the potential to make predictions about known and unknown elements. The same holds true for the elements' use in homeopathy, where the essence of each remedy reflects their chemical properties, revealing the healing power found in nature.

Homeopaths have applied Scholten's concept of stages successfully, first with the mineral remedies and more recently with the plant remedies, according to their chemical composition. The theory provides a way of associating what a person does, and how they react in certain situations, with the simillimum.

The remedy I had been taking, *Samarium phosphoricum*, was a stage eight remedy. That fact, in the light of my colleague's comment that it was completely understandable that the eighth chapter should be the most difficult, led me to understand that the chapters of this book correspond to the first ten stages of the elements. This, the eighth chapter, pulls together all the ideas I've so far presented so that the selection of case stories in Chapter 9 makes sense, and is fully realised and understood. Thereafter a reader can successfully reach Chapter 10, the summit.

Mindfulness

Somewhere along my own journey, a shift occurred, and experiences with homeopathy expanded my previously orthodox world view. The explanation as to how that happened is rather simple, and pertains to our ability to be open to new experiences and possibilities. We change, grow, and develop most effectively in a state of non-judgemental curiosity. This can be likened to a childlike state of awareness in which we observe what *is*, rather than what our programmed thoughts and beliefs tell us *should be*. This state is often referred to as *mindfulness*; in it, we are fully present in the moment, and have a capacity for expansion and acceptance of what might otherwise be too uncomfortable. It provides us with an opportunity to fully experience ourselves and our environment.

Age-old concepts of mindfulness have recently been taken on by those working in the fields of psychology and health. Evidence for the health benefits of practising this state within our daily lives has rapidly accumulated. A book I have been recommending, *The Happiness Trap* (2007), by GP Dr Russ Harris, explores the concept, and is easy to read and re-read. My own experiences and observations have shown me that this state of awareness and clarity – of seeing ourselves and the world as it truly is – can occur spontaneously as part of a positive response to a well-chosen homeopathic remedy.

Throughout our lives, our beliefs shape our experiences, which in turn have the capacity to shape our beliefs, forming a feedback loop in a progressive spiral, as illustrated in Figure 2.

Time for a new world view

I believe that there needs to be wider acceptance of a whole-person approach within the field of medicine in general.

My rediscovery of homeopathy, after having first read about it years earlier, resulted in many new experiences, as I opened up to what amounts to a new world view. I have since heard many stories similar to my own, of medical doctors studying homeopathy after a personal healing experience, and developing a new world view accordingly.

The first step in the process is recognising that we each hold a world view: a belief system through which we see and experience everything. It acts like a filter through which we perceive life. Ultimately, this world view creates and therefore limits our reality.

The next step in the path to a new, expanded world view lies in the paradigm shift necessary for change. Before we engage in any process of change, we first need to acknowledge the need for it.

Figure 2: The spiral of experiences and beliefs

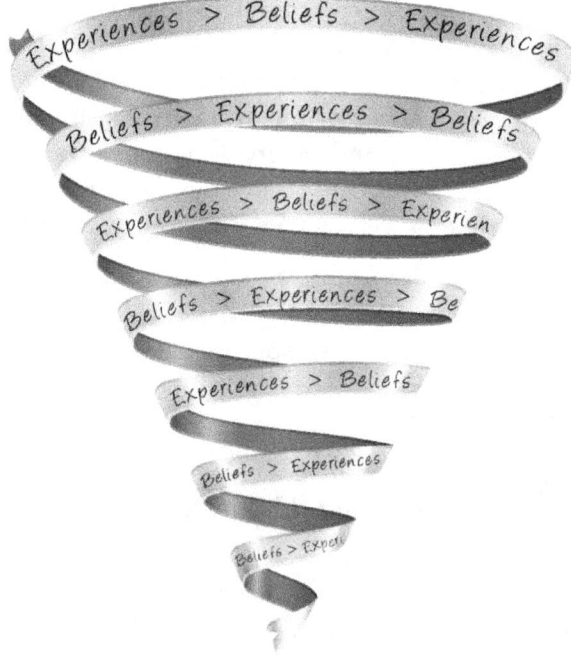

The problem: a crisis in healthcare

Years of experience in general practice have shown me change is overdue. The limited world view provided by the bio-medical model sets doctors up to fail, and creates unrealistic expectations among the public. It seems as if patient-centred care has been overtaken by increasingly disease-centred research, as we look to technology for a "cure" for the human condition. Health and pharmaceutical budgets can't keep up with rising costs and rising demands. In New Zealand we face a health crisis as a result of our aging population. At the same time, in our technologically driven medical system, there is ever more specialisation and sub-specialisation; doctors are trained with extra expertise in various body parts or body systems. We acknowledge these doctors as specialists and hold them in high regard, but the progressive lack of integration this system entails means that at the individual patient level the whole person is at risk of being overlooked.

Trained as generalists, general practitioners have the ideal opportunity to focus on whole-person care, but sadly the medical system isn't geared toward rewarding doctors for spending time with patients. The extra cost such a shift in priority would entail may not be affordable for people, or they may not see value in spending more time with a practitioner. Economic pressures affect patients and doctors alike, pushing us toward a regime characterised by multiple short appointments tending to focus on prescription medication as the solution. The tradition and benefit of doctors listening to patients is undervalued and at risk of being lost.

Compliance requirements by health funding authorities demand increasing accountability on the part of doctors for the outcomes of various chronic diseases in patient populations. These health outcomes are chosen for ease of measurability, so they focus on numbers. Meanwhile, high rates of diabetes, cardiovascular disease, and obesity are fuelled by the easy availability and intensive advertising of high-fat, high-calorie fast foods by big business. These expanding problems, along with growing levels of child poverty, were very much the focus of the New Zealand General Practice Conference I attended most recently, in 2014. Although the problems have been identified, effective solutions so far have not. I believe that the solutions require a new way of seeing the whole picture.

The solution: a four-cornered approach

Medicine didn't evolve in a vacuum – it continues to develop along with the human condition. As individuals and groups we develop in paradigm shifts, moving through progressive stages of awareness. Modern philosophers continue to seek answers and models for these shifts, as Socrates did long ago.

American philosopher Ken Wilber suggests that while the rational-industrial world view brought many important changes, including the end of slavery; equal rights for women; and advances in science, art, and medicine, the next step is to be open to modes of consciousness that transcend or move beyond industrialisation (Wilber, 2000). Human progress or evolution always includes, incorporates, and then goes beyond (*transcends*) the earlier situation, whatever that may be.

Both Wilber and Sheldrake use the concept of *holons* and *holarchies,* as originally described by Arthur Koestler, to provide a framework to understand our reality and describe the natural interconnection between all things. A *holon* is any entity that in itself is a whole, yet is also part of some greater whole. The utility of this simple concept becomes clear as we see that it applies to *everything*. There are natural hierarchies of increasing wholeness, and everything is a *holon*; the word *holarchy* describes this inclusive evolutionary process of increasing wholeness.

Wilber explains that there is a common evolutionary thread of *holarchy*, running from *matter* to *life* to *mind* to *spirit*. All together these elements form what Wilber describes as the *Kosmos*. He uses the Greek spelling to indicate that the concept also involves *spirit*, since "cosmos" is often used to apply only to the physical universe. In the process of transcending and including what has gone before, evolution has an overall direction or tendency to move toward increasing complexity through differentiation, organisation, and autonomy. Wilber defines *spirit* as an increasing spectrum of consciousness: an immense intelligence of which we are all a part, in a process of moving from *subconscious* to *self-conscious* to *super-conscious* (oneness). Because each step always transcends and includes, in a process of unfolding and enfolding, *spirit* is found in each step. Wilber explains, therefore, that *spirit* cannot be separated from *matter*, *life*, or *mind*, and started with the very beginning, which Wilber describes as the "Emptiness", before the "Big Bang".

Seeking the common ground in hundreds of developmental maps from all over the world, in historical and modern times, Wilber realised they needed to be accommodated in four different areas. He describes these as the Four Corners of the Kosmos, as shown here in Figure 3. The left side refers to the *subjective/inside experience*, and the right side refers to the *objective/outside view*. The top half is about the *individual* and the bottom half the *collective*. This creates four quadrants. Most importantly, all four quadrants are interconnected and mutually interdependent.

The relevance of this conceptual model to medicine becomes clear as we compare and differentiate the *objective view from outside* with *subjective experience or meaning from inside* (the story). Wilber says that "Spirit exists in and as all four quadrants," so any further human transformation requires an integral approach including all four quadrants. He goes on to show how these four quadrants can be further simplified as the big three – "I", "we", "it" – the areas of life in which spirit manifests.

Figure 3: The four quadrants

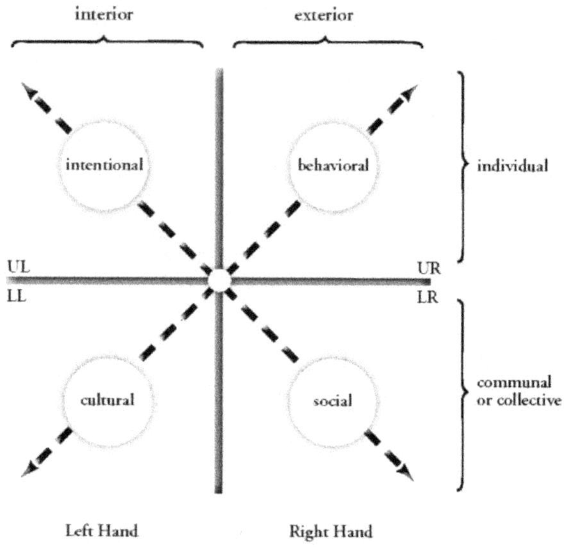

From *A Brief History of Everything*, by Ken Wilber, ©1996 by Ken Wilber. Reprinted by arrangement with Shambhala Publications, Inc., Boston, www.shambhala.com

While orthodox medicine is currently somewhat restricted to the exterior or right-sided quadrants, homeopathy acknowledges all four. We know the right-side objective viewpoint of orthodox medicine works as far as it goes, but in this regard I find relevant Wilber's concern that often the very existence of "I" and "we" are denied. Wilber warns also how, as individuals, we can isolate ourselves, becoming stuck in a limited view of spirit represented only in the upper left quadrant, as "I", focusing only on the self, and denying the other quadrants.

Wilber predicts that the paradigm shift already under way, transcending and including progress already made, will involve both a change in consciousness and a change in institutions, to encompass a balanced four-quadrant integral world view:

> In medicine, for example, you can see that any effective care would have to take into account, not just the objective medicine or physical treatment that you give the person (UR), but also the person's subjective beliefs and expectations (UL), the cultural attitudes, hopes and fears about sickness (LL), and the social institutions, economic factors and access to health care (LR), all of which have a causal effect on the course of a person's illness (because all four quadrants cause, and are caused by, the others) (Wilber, 2000, p. 310).

Homeopathy and the four corners

Homeopathy, through its focus on individualisation, takes an all four-quadrant approach. Because homeopathy treats the *person* – not the diagnosis or disease, which is not a necessary step toward finding the simillimum – it doesn't standalone in situations when a diagnosis is desirable and all the treatment options, including allopathic, are being considered. Historically, there was no need for a diagnosis, when the physiology of the human body wasn't comprehended and the priority was to treat safely and effectively. In modern times our increasing knowledge makes it more relevant to obtain this information through the traditional medical process, combining history, examination and appropriate diagnostic tests, which allow treatment options to then be fully explored.

As a medical doctor, I believe homeopathy has its place alongside orthodox medicine. Registered homeopaths have undergone training in the medical sciences to ensure they have the capacity to practise safely and appropriately; they know when to refer their clients to a doctor for further assessment. The current medical system is deficient in the left quadrants, where homeopathy is strong, and homeopaths do not compete in the right quadrants, where orthodox medicine is able to provide objective medical assessment and diagnosis. A combined collaborative approach opens up exciting possibilities for healing.

The change under way

Homeopaths are not alone in their frustration with the limitations of the currently accepted paradigm of medicine. Other medical doctors are speaking up, and questioning the widely accepted bio-medical model of disease. Already I have referred to ground-breaking work by Dr Brian Broom, an honorary lecturer at Auckland University, which now offers a mind–body diploma course to health professionals. Dr Robin Kelly had a background in general practice when he began practising acupuncture. He had been impressed by the safety and effectiveness of this ancient Chinese healing art, and went on to study its roots in traditional Chinese medicine. He has since published two books about healing in the mind–body paradigm, *The Human Antenna* (2008) and *The Human Hologram* (2011).

Experience tells me there is no shortage of empathetic caring doctors and other professionals we can really count on who work diligently and quietly to provide wonderful healthcare. The problem lies within the prevailing medical system, which is adherent to an outdated philosophy originating from historical times. Recognising this, anaesthetist Dr Robin Youngson recently set up a global network, Hearts in Healthcare, with the intention of "re-humanising" healthcare for the benefit of health professionals and their patients: "to support, generate and facilitate compassionate care in the healthcare system". He points out that, historically, the industrialisation of healthcare dehumanised the system. His book Time to Care (2012) courageously exposes the shocking realities often hidden within the medical system;

those of us indoctrinated into this system can easily identify with these realities. The book suggests healthier ways to treat ourselves and others, supported by two hundred references supporting Youngson's ideas about the significance of compassion. Youngson's philosophy is summarised in his statement, "Healthcare's focus on physical disease and bio-medicine is unbalanced. We need to pay much more attention to emotional, psychological and spiritual wellbeing and the huge importance of healing relationships."

Conclusion

There is a pattern emerging. The Kosmos is a multidimensional quantum field, of which we are all an important part. Many great thinkers, describing the phenomenology of life, have reached similar conclusions. Sheldrake's hypothesis of morphogenic fields in biology, for example, accounts for the same concepts of partness and wholeness, where like influences like across space and time. Observing synchronicity, Jung referred to his experiences of a similar interconnecting field of information, recognisable in both inner and outer dimensions. Hahnemann saw the same process in action, observing that a person's symptoms often indicated the substance they needed, leading to the guiding principle of homeopathy, "let likes be cured with likes".

The healing power of story is revealed in the next chapter, which presents real cases from my homeopathic consultations.

CHAPTER NINE

From Story to Substance

The three cases I discuss in this chapter represent a very small sample of the breadth of cases I've taken over the years. I've chosen them to demonstrate the various sources of homeopathic remedies, with substances from the animal, mineral, and plant kingdoms.

I am most grateful to those who gave permission for their personal illness experiences to be shared here for the benefit of others. I've changed their identifying details in these stories, to protect confidentiality.

Homeopathic care for chronic conditions is completely individualised. At the initial consultation, neither practitioner nor patient knows where the story will lead. Unlike in orthodox medicine, there is no set formula or therapeutic programme for consultation and treatment to follow, and outcomes cannot be guaranteed based on statistics. The process is more like embarking on a journey, intending to arrive at a destination of "cure" or resolution of symptoms: the exact route and travel time is never known at the outset.

Responses to remedies for chronic problems vary from sudden and dramatic to slow and subtle. Results don't always show in the first few days or even weeks. When you decide to "give homeopathy a try", you should know that success depends on you as well as the practitioner. The therapeutic relationship is really a partnership: be willing to engage in a process of self-discovery on the path to healing. Those little pills or drops are a powerful catalyst, allowing your body's own innate intelligence to do the rest.

Oliver: *Hyoscyamusniger* (plant, nightshade family, "henbane")

A concerned mother brought her six-year-old son, Oliver, to see me about his challenging behaviour and his loose bowel motions. She felt both were caused by oversensitivity to physical, mental and emotional stimulation. Assessment by a child psychologist placed Oliver on the spectrum of Asperger's syndrome, part of a group of medical diagnoses called autistic spectrum disorder. His mother had engaged in the "Incredible Years" programme for parents with children aged three to eight years and had found it beneficial, but Oliver's behaviour didn't improve.

Oliver was intelligent, and enjoyed learning. He was fully focused on tasks, often so engaged that he resisted change, becoming disruptive in class. Play times were a major challenge for Oliver and his family: the company of more than two children resulted in too much stimulation. His behaviour was unpredictable, and could suddenly change and deteriorate. He would become physically agitated, shouting and jumping, waving his arms around, and spinning as if trying to create some personal space. The lashing out included scratching or clawing motions and was indiscriminate: anyone too close could get hurt. At these times Oliver was completely out of control: his mother described him as "crazy, laughing like a hyena". Understandably, several parents made complaints to the school when their children were injured or upset.

Oliver's mum didn't think Oliver meant to be violent. He disliked competition and aggression, but if others were aggressive, or if he was punished, he responded in the same way. He spent hours absorbed in play with insects and spiders, making homes for them, and never harming or hurting them. He didn't play rough with his younger brother, who adored him, but Oliver tended to withdraw from his brother and limit his physical contact with him, preferring to play alone. In contrast, he often sought cuddles from Mum, asking to be tickled, and giggling uncontrollably.

The major behaviour problems had started when Oliver was just two and a half years old. His mother recounted circumstances that had caused extreme stress for her at the time his little brother was born, and described how overwhelmed she had felt. Oliver had wanted attention constantly, demanding it by physically attacking his mother, and there were problems with aggression at preschool. Oliver's behaviour was always worse when he ate sugary foods, which he loved. Ice cream worsened his diarrhoea. His motions were always loose, and he had several daily, but when he was upset or overstimulated he would feel a sudden urge and just "let go", resulting in episodes of incontinence.

Oliver's general health was good, with the occasional respiratory or ear infection from time to time. His childhood immunisation programme had started late, after he had turned three, and there was no sign of any adverse reaction to it. Mental health problems, particularly mood-regulation issues and substance abuse, featured strongly in Oliver's family history.

Oliver's mother thought she'd suffered in the past from postnatal depression, saying that she hadn't felt "a real connection" after Oliver was born by elective caesarean section. Oliver had been breastfed for six months, and reached his milestones at age-appropriate times, crawling at great speed and walking by fourteen months. As a baby, Oliver would startle easily to noise, flinging his arms out on either side, as if for protection. He was very sensitive to separation, and disliked being left at preschool.

Oliver's mother observed that Oliver "exudes heat", and that his behaviour was generally much worse when he was overheated, with "a red face and sweaty head". He coped better in cool environments. Oliver's mother was constantly "trying to keep him and his body in perfect equilibrium". She tried hard to maintain routines, which helped, but if Oliver was hungry or tired, his behaviour rapidly deteriorated. Swimming was one of Oliver's favourite activities. He was "amazing in water," his mother said: "he spends the whole time under water, being a fish". In contrast, on land, his style of running and movement appeared poorly coordinated.

The first remedy I gave to Oliver was a mineral, *Magnesium carbonicum* 200c. It's commonly needed by a child who responds with anxiety to a situation of conflict between parents, or the absence of one or both parents; this leads to withdrawal or aggression. Such children commonly experience a feeling of abandonment and a need for the security of extra care and protection. *Mag carb* matched Oliver's general symptoms, and initially he did very well with this remedy, but over several months the benefits noticeably lessened. After that, Oliver's mother attended follow-up consultations without bringing Oliver along, because being the centre of attention was another trigger for Oliver's aggressive behaviour. During this time Oliver's family were waiting to enter the multidisciplinary assessment process at the local hospital, to receive extra support.

Lessening of the effects of repeat doses of homeopathy over time indicates palliation (temporary relief of symptoms) rather than cure (resolution of symptoms). I changed the remedy to *Magnesium phosphoricum* because the element *Phosphorus* relates to contact and communication with peers, which seemed more specific for Oliver's aggression; this significantly reduced Oliver's aggression.

At this point, Oliver's mother told me: "The hard-core aggression is gone. The behaviour's more positive, but still intense". Oliver's teachers had been commenting that Oliver was better in the playground; he was "not hitting and scratching". Oliver's mother had noticed more "internal heat":

Oliver would have "a bright red face after school". His behaviour now was characterised by "silliness", with "a hyena laugh, a red face, craziness and stupidity". "It's extreme happiness," his mother told me: "he just loves laughing. He's even more silly with other kids, there's lots of toilet talk, poos and bums and bum holes".

I needed to know more, so I asked Oliver's mother directly, "Has Oliver ever had any tendency to expose himself – I mean his genital area?" His mother answered with a sigh of relief: "Oh my God, yes!" She went on to tell me that Oliver had seemed "highly sexualised since he was a baby". He was masturbating more as he grew older, particularly when he was upset. His cuddles were difficult for Oliver's mother because the way he touched her body felt inappropriate, like she was being groped. We agreed that children are naturally inclined to explore their bodies and genitals from a young age, but Oliver's mother felt this focus of his behaviour was getting much worse. Her conversations with the mothers of boys the same age indicated Oliver's behaviour was extreme. Recently, on returning to her car after running an errand, Oliver's mother had found Oliver in the car standing at the window laughing, exposing his genitals to people in the street passing by.

I now realised the remedy this child needed was *Hyoscyamus*, made from a plant from the *Solanaceae* family, which includes the remedies *Belladonna* (deadly nightshade), and *Stramonium* (datura). The essence of *Hyoscyamus* is a feeling of being let down, deserted, or betrayed by the person on whom one is completely dependent. The initial response is trying to attract attention by ridiculous silly behaviour. Eventually this can escalate to violence from feeling persecuted, which forces others to take notice. Usually, but not always, this is a "hyper-sexual" remedy. The proving symptoms include elements of shamelessness and exhibitionism, great restlessness, mood disturbances, and often jealousy. All these elements were present in this case: Oliver's behavioural problem escalated immediately after the birth of his younger brother, when he wanted more attention. Oliver suffered from "involuntary stool from excitement", another symptom of the remedy. The family, *Solanaceae*, shares his symptoms of heat and facial flushing.

I gave Oliver *Hyoscyamus* 200c, instructing his mother to give him two doses a few hours apart. After Oliver took this remedy, there was a noticeable improvement in his behaviour within just a few days. He began dealing with challenging and excitable moments much better. He could now cope with noisy group environments such as birthday parties, where many children were present, and the problems at school disappeared. Oliver's mum gave him a further dose of the remedy about a month later, when Oliver again began to have short-lived bursts of anger, and the remedy settled the behaviour. With great relief, she told me: "The whole sexuality thing is gone, the groping is gone, and the exhibitionism is gone!" Naturally, Oliver continued to be a very creative, high-energy child: this was his nature. However, periodic doses of *Hyoscyamus* reduced his tendency to overly sexual behaviour and prevented him from becoming uncontrollably silly or aggressive, so he remained focused at school.

Graeme: *Erbium muriaticum* (lanthanide mineral)

Graeme attended a long homeopathic consultation some years ago, just before his fiftieth birthday. He'd been diagnosed with depression, leading to several years of psychotherapy. After the therapy Graeme understood the origins of his problem, but his mood wasn't improving. The first antidepressant he had been prescribed did not alter his mood, and another had quickly resulted in suicidal thoughts, so it was stopped.

Graeme's problems had all started soon after his father died when Graeme was a teenager. He said that at this time "life was bleak and grim, as if everything was black and white. There was no colour." He described "a sensation of brushing up against something strong like a dam, with some flexibility perhaps; it seemed not possible, a light on the other side". Through therapy, Graeme came to realise that "my mother was an extremely controlling woman. I grew up in a controlled protestant repressive small country town with no social life. I was not heard as a child and my emotional needs were not met; I was even dressed by her." He recalled of his childhood: "There were no books, no culture. I was starved; nourishment was lacking. I felt dull and despairing." Graeme married young, and thereafter stayed many years in a "no-touch relationship", in which he "felt obliged to bring up the kids".

Graeme went to university to explore his own creativity and become a writer; he said: "It was the first thing I ever did for myself." Graeme's feeling of being beside a "wall" had lasted many years. "I think about the other side and how it would feel," he related: "I have a sense of the rest of me being on the other side where it's light. Here I feel flat, empty, deadness, dullness, heavy. What's the point of living this life, yet to be fulfilled? It's existential despair."

Graeme was a solitary child; even now, he felt that he had too little contact with others. He described his father as a workaholic who had died unexpectedly from over-work. Graeme had loved him dearly, but never cried after his death; he said that he had been taught not to have feelings. Graeme smoked cannabis to help motivate his work, and felt it made life bearable, as a way of blocking things out. However, he resented the fact that he used it as a crutch. In the past, he had used other drugs, "as an investigation of consciousness". Graeme had always been interested in the occult, alchemy and astrology. He said "I am interested in the hidden side of life." He told me that there had been periods in his life when he had experienced inertia: "I can't do anything; it's like I am completely not there or I cease to exist, with no feeling, like a shell, and hours go by." Graeme had had suicidal ideas during these "unfeeling times", but had felt he wouldn't carry it through, as he felt a deep spiritual need to finish at some point.

Graeme's past history had included occasional respiratory infections and migraine headaches. He had a background of long-term smoking. He had suffered orchitis (inflammation of the testes) with the mumps in his early teens, and had spent a few weeks in hospital as a young baby after being "starved" during a gastroenteritis illness.

Graeme was upset by injustice, particularly toward children, because he had felt powerless as a child, and recalled from his childhood "a horrible fear of needles" that had started with his first vaccination.

There was no apparent response to the first remedy I recommended to Graeme, *Cannabis indica* 200c (cannabis), so I chose another, *Lac maternum* 200c (breast milk). Two months later Graeme reported: "I have turned the corner; a bit like a click, it's great". He had realised he needed to move away from his elderly mother to gain more personal space, and felt comfortable with this decision. I did not see Graeme again until a couple of years later, when he reported his mood to be mostly normal with some ups and downs. At that point I gave a further dose of the remedy.

Several years later, Graeme attended a homeopathic follow-up appointment, and reported feeling ready to commit suicide. He had explored methods to end his own life. He felt "empty hollowed-outness", an "absence of feeling", and "numbness, not sadness". He told me: "I can achieve only with great effort; there's nothing else I want to do." Only awareness of the impact his death would have on his loved ones was stopping him from committing suicide. He described the feeling as follows: "I recede into myself naturally. From childhood I learned the world won't support you – to not have expectations. The outside can't be trusted."

The remedy I gave at this point was a mineral from the Lanthanide series of the periodic table, *Cerium oxydatum* 200c. I had recently learned about this group of homeopathic remedies at a seminar with Jan Scholten. The group shares the theme of responsibility for self, seeking autonomy, and self-exploration, encompassing the "shadow side". Themes of the remedy *Cerium* include a lack of confidence; a feeling of being enclosed or cocooned. The remedy *Oxygen* (oxydatum) is associated with the feeling of being abused, often with indignation.

We met for a follow-up appointment just after the catastrophic 2011 tsunami in Japan.

Graeme told me that he remained depressed, and that he'd been exploring euthanasia online. Our conversation turned to the tsunami. I recall an image developing in my own mind of a black wall of water as Graeme spoke. He said: "seeing it on television, it feels like Armageddon accelerating: an apocalypse". Graeme went on to talk of contempt for his mother, and for the place he now lived. He wanted access to a cosmopolitan city, possibly East Berlin, as he loved intellectual stimulation, learning, and new ideas. He said: "here is a vacuum, no air. I am invisible; I do need the world to respond to me in some way." Graeme still felt that he was "in a dark place: no doors, no light, just hopelessness." In response to my promise to get back to him with a new remedy, he said: "There's no hurry. It's not urgent; my life is boring."

Now I gave Graeme *Erbium muriaticum* 200c, a different lanthanide salt, because I saw that the tsunami, the black wall of water, resonated with the patient and this remedy. Remarkably, the wall Graeme had described, with the feeling of separation, has an association with *Erbium*. In *Secret Lanthanides* (2005), Jan Scholten refers to the famous album by

Pink Floyd, *The Wall*: this also represents a direct link with Berlin, which Graeme had mentioned. *Erbium* matches the drug-taking culture of the song "Comfortably Numb", expressing a feeling of emptiness and powerlessness leading to resignation and gloom. *Muriaticum* (chloride) represents a lack of nurturing, care and mother.

After taking the remedy, Graeme reported "feelings of lightness"; he no longer had thoughts of "hopelessness". He became more productive at work, and his energy improved. He developed a recurrence of bronchitis, but did not take antibiotics this time, and it resolved by itself. Graeme made plans to travel and "redefine" himself. I received occasional updates from him by email until we met at a GP appointment well over a year later. At that point he was fit and well and had improved blood pressure; he had also lost some excess weight.

Barbara: *Apis mellifica* (honey bee poison)

Barbara was sixty-two when she booked a GP appointment with me to find out if homeopathy could help her. She was "feeling frantic", experiencing intense itching in her anal area: "like worms wriggling". The symptoms had started eight to ten years earlier, she said. She felt as if the doctors must think her crazy, as nothing seemed to help. She had taken many worm treatments over the years, she told me. She had developed anal splits and soreness after passing hard bowel motions, but she had also experienced diarrhoea when she was anxious, resulting in a diagnosis of irritable bowel syndrome. On examination, I noted inflammation surrounding the anus, with spots and small fissures in the skin. Later, at the initial homeopathic consultation, she told me: "it causes a pulsation – like three thousand worms screwing around in there."

I observed Barbara fidget and move frequently around on her chair; she leaned forward as she spoke. She was open and direct. She spoke quickly, with intensity, and made plenty of eye contact. Her cheeks were red. Later, at the first follow-up consultation, I wondered if her voice had a "buzzing" quality.

Her anal symptoms had first started in childhood, she told me, when she'd had "worms". Although she'd often been constipated during her teens, she also got diarrhoea from anxiety, usually during changes in her routine. This was a recurring problem. She recalled the embarrassment of having worms. As a teenager, she had fallen ill with a kidney problem, and had been kept in bed for about two months; the doctor had visited daily.

Barbara had a history of food allergies. She got hives from pineapple juice, and once became breathless, with hives and facial swelling, after eating cauliflower. Barbara was taking an antihistamine tablet every day to control her symptoms. She described having had "chronic vaginal thrush" that was "very itchy, raw and sore" in all her pregnancies, saying that it "nearly drove me mental!" Her other health problems included high blood pressure, reflux of gastric acid, post-menopausal hot flushes, and coughing since a bout of double pneumonia, which she had treated with asthma inhalers. To control these symptoms, Barbara was taking regular medication for her blood pressure, and to suppress her stomach acid, in addition to hormone replacement therapy (HRT) to control her hot flushes.

At work, Barbara described herself as very busy – she couldn't stop running, and was "fast and thorough": "I just go like my foot's on the accelerator into a job; full pelt ahead!" She acknowledged that work had been an important part of her childhood; she'd often been required to help in the family business, including working on public holidays. She said "I just love working, and cleaning", explaining how this had annoyed her husband and caused conflict early in their marriage. Barbara's home was immaculate, and she loved to work in the garden. She had a strong sense of loyalty and respect for her parents, her husband, and her employer. While Barbara considered herself to be open and trusting, by her own admission she would "get angry and blow up" when she was criticised. She told me: "if someone shits on me I'm gutted! I lose sleep and I'm offended". A family dispute had resulted in a complete loss of contact with her daughter for many years.

Barbara confided to me that although she probably came across to others as confident, she felt "very inferior": "I am hopeless at spelling, and avoid writing, but I can talk and communicate". She felt ashamed about her lack of skill with language, and told me that in the past she had been so terrified of reading out loud that the anticipation had caused episodes of sudden dysentery. She said that her children had experienced similar reading problems. Barbara disliked travel, preferring the "security of home and routine", and expressed a fear of flying over the sea. She had "a shocking fear of water – I won't swim". She also told me of her fear of wetas, recalling that she had once nearly fainted during an encounter with one. However, she also expressed a love of animals, saying that she kept many pets, and liked to feed the birds in her garden.

After hearing Barbara's case I didn't immediately know what remedy to give, although I suspected the simillimum belonged to the animal kingdom. I undertook formal repertorisation using computer software designed for the purpose, but this didn't reveal a likely choice, so I looked at possible animal remedies and chose *Apis mellifica* because it fitted the central complaint: intense itching. Barbara's agitation, desire to be busy, and work constantly suited this remedy. Her allergic reactions, including hives and facial swelling, are prominent proving symptoms of *Apis*, and the remedy picture includes asthma. The kidney illness Barbara had suffered from in her teens may have been glomerulonephritis, which can affect kidney function, fluid balance, and blood pressure, all symptoms associated with *Apis*. The way Barbara spoke, using forceful, sometimes "coarse" language, along with sudden flare-ups of anger, matched the remedy. Feeling stupid and inferior is a common symptom associated with insect remedies and the animal kingdom generally. Other symptoms associated with the remedy *Apis* are heat and intensity, matching Barbara's hot flushes, her intensity of symptoms, and her appearance of red cheeks. Later, during a follow-up consultation, Barbara mentioned that both her brother and her daughter experienced anaphylaxis from bee stings.

I gave Barbara only a couple of doses of *Apis* 200c. After this, she told me that the itching was a lot better. It had nearly resolved when I saw her five weeks later.

Barbara told me that the throbbing irritation was gone. She commented that she was feeling "more calm"; this was confirmed by changes in her appearance and manner. A further six weeks later there was no itching at all, and Barbara said: "I am feeling like my batteries are recharged, I have much more energy." A few months later Barbara began to slowly reduce the antihistamine tablets she had been taking, and stopped using asthma inhalers. Two years later her cough was minimal and she was taking only one or two HRT tablets per week, but she remained on the acid-suppressing medicine a specialist had advised her to take. She also continued to take a very small dose of beta-blocker medication, after experiencing heart palpitations when she had stopped taking it.

Conclusion

When I am approached by people considering homeopathy, I am frequently asked whether I have experience treating their particular disease or problem with homeopathy. Unfortunately, my attempts to explain that homeopathy treats the person rather than the disease are often met with scepticism and doubt, because orthodox medicine is disease-oriented.

These three cases explore the whole-person experiences of three very different individuals, with very different problems. The simillimum found in each case was very different too – the remedies I've discussed here are only a small sample of the spectrum of homeopathic remedies. However, these stories share a simple, powerful message – the need for the health practitioner to look at a person's whole story.

CHAPTER TEN

Reaching Balance and Harmony

"I am the Lorax. I speak for the trees. I speak for the trees, for the trees have no tongues."

Dr Seuss, The Lorax

Homeopathy and orthodox medicine side by side

In the preceding chapters I have shared my experience as a doctor encountering homeopathy as a completely new and unfamiliar concept, leading to my current understanding of the philosophy and science surrounding this remarkable system of healing. From the beginning I knew homeopathy didn't fit comfortably within the orthodox bio-medical system, but that it was consistent with my earliest understanding of mind–body medicine, developed during GP training in patient-centred whole-person care.

The unity of the mind–body method works much like an invisible interconnecting web or network, binding together seemingly separate symptoms, sensations, and disease processes to describe a person's whole experience. We already know that linear theories of causation provide an inadequate explanation of these complex acausal – yet meaningful – associations. In a mind–body approach, a healer must fully appreciate this unity; in order to find the most suitable treatment, he or she must take a step back, to observe the whole person.

There are many mind–body treatment options, but I prefer homeopathy, with its integrated system of therapy resulting in remedy choices that are safe and efficacious.

I spent ten years attempting to combine the two methodologies – orthodox bio-medicine and homeopathy – under one roof. It led me only to frustration and fatigue. I came to realise that fulfilling my role as an effective GP allowed me little opportunity to reflect on the bigger, whole-person picture for individual patients, and explore possible solutions with them. People often present with multiple problems, and the need to formulate confident diagnoses while practising safe medicine and maintaining the necessary documentation inevitably results in the squeeze of time pressure. It is always difficult for doctors working in this environment to stand back and view the whole situation. For this reason, I came to see a place for homeopathy operating respectfully alongside, rather than integrated or absorbed within, orthodox medicine.

Posing the question

About a year ago, and a year after starting this book project, I attended a five-day homeopathy retreat in the beautiful Waitakere Ranges with internationally renowned homeopath and teacher Alize Timmerman.

At the start of the seminar, after the introductions were over, Alize asked us to reflect on why we were here. My reflection took the form of a question: How could I share the valuable medical knowledge, skills, and experience I'd gathered over the years most effectively with more patients, and more people? Over the course of the seminar, I participated in a group proving of *Rimu* that provided an answer to this difficult question, propelling me closer to my achievement of a long-term goal.

I share this story to demonstrate the potential of homeopathy as a method of facilitating progress, evolution, and healing not only for individuals or families, but also for wider groups of people. This tenth chapter represents the summit, or homeopathy's "Stage 10". At the summit, a much wider view becomes possible. Those working in the field of homeopathy are already well aware of such potential, and many more provings are being undertaken to investigate and understand the potential for healing using homeopathic preparations of natural substances, including the large kingdom of plants.

The *Rimu* proving

Alize is from the Netherlands. For this seminar in New Zealand, she wanted the group to choose an indigenous tree from which to carry out a *proving by trituration*. The process would be different to Hahnemann's traditional method of ingesting a substance potentised in solution; it would involve grinding a small amount of a substance with milk sugar in a mortar and pestle, and then carrying out serial dilution using more milk sugar. Eventually we decided to use a rimu tree growing close by. We spent an hour of the first afternoon grinding bark and fresh leaf into powder, according to guidelines found in *The Trituration Handbook* (Hogeland & Schriebman, 2008). Alize told us to particularly note any physical sensations, thoughts, or feelings we became aware of throughout the process, and to take care to write them down.

After the first round of trituration was completed, we undertook an interesting exercise in pairs, making use of the proving notes we'd all made. One partner had to form a phrase or sentence of no more than five words for the other, using that person's proving notes. The first person then had to repeatedly whisper this phrase into one ear of the second person, while a third person joined the pair to whisper into the other ear. I heard the reassuring words "Group supports enthusiastic harmony" again and again, and felt as if the words were revealing the beginning of an answer to my question.

Half of this seminar involved Alize sharing her vast knowledge with us, presenting cases and themes of interest. The remaining half involved our immersion in the proving process. Over just a few days, I noticed two processes of change occurring. We took turns sharing our individual personal experiences; as one person shared the insights he or she had gained from dreams, symptoms, and sensations, others would inevitably identify with particular aspects of the "story", and offer similar insights. At the same time, the group formed a cohesive whole, undergoing what seemed like a collective process of change.

I wondered how it could be that our group experienced so much of the information of *Rimu*, simply from carrying out the trituration together.

During the trituration process, as the rimu was ground in a mortar and pestle with lactose powder, a cloud of fine dust arose. It was barely visible hanging in the air, but noticeable on re-entering the room. Hanging our heads directly over our bowls, we breathed both the substance and the powder at each stage of the grinding and progressive dilution. The moist, sensitive mucous membranes lining our upper respiratory tracts provided an ideal method of absorption. Somehow, this process allowed us to interact with and experience the substance at a quantum-energy level.

Synchronicity in the *Rimu* proving

By the third day I was longing to get out of the room into the fresh air and enjoy the bush. When an opportunity arose to escape, I took a long, energising walk in light rain, discovering many beautiful spaces beneath the trees. At one point I felt a faint "plop" against my raincoat, but looking down I saw only leaves. Later, in the bathroom mirror, I discovered that one of my silver hoop earrings was missing. By then I couldn't recall which particular tree I had stopped under, and my attempts to retrace my steps proved futile.

Earrings are my favourite piece of jewellery. I feel undressed without them. Strangely, the only other earring I had ever lost was from a similar pair of silver hoops; it had fallen off on a walk around the base track of Mauao back home. I had been unable to find it again, but had easily replaced it with this new set. The synchronicity of losing one earring from the new pair was hard to miss. This time I felt that somehow I had been fooled, and had paid the price to the bush and the trees. The essence of *Rimu* was unfolding during the proving, and themes of trickery and sacrifice were part of the story (see below).

Circle, spiral, and vortex shapes featured as key symbols during the proving of *Rimu*. Once during the process, I glanced down at the mortar in my lap and noticed a perfect spiral had formed in the powder. I shrugged it off, assuming that grinding in a round bowl could easily produce such a shape. But when I tried to recreate the effect, I could not. The spiral is related to the "concha", a shell shape similar to that found in our ears. Symptoms relating to the ear were prominent during our proving. On the fourth evening of trituration the group started to "sing", forming harmonious vocal sounds. This caused intense persistent pain deep in my right ear. When the pain subsided I tried to join in, but couldn't make a sound. However, a short time later I found my voice, joining the harmonious wordless song filling the room.

Rimu: themes

I have extracted the main themes of the trituration proving we undertook as a group from my personal proving notes and experiences shared by the group, as the full collation of the group proving information was not yet available at the time of writing.

> *Themes of Rimu**
>
> Individual <-> Group
>
> Connection <-> Disconnection, Separation
>
> Enthusiasm <-> Indifference
>
> Co-operation <-> Competition, Abuse
>
> Harmony <-> Chaos
>
> Ritual, Rules, System, Sacrifice <-> Freedom
>
> Birth, Renewal <-> Death, Destruction
>
> Earth, Underground <-> Sky, Heaven
>
> Babies, Children <-> History, Ancestry and Indigenous People
>
> Symbols: Circle, Spiral, Vortex, Silver
>
> Animal: Bird
>
> Physical: Head, ears, eyes, nose, vision, hearing, throat, voice, limbs, uterus, skin
>
> Sensations: Spinning, flying, falling, floating, fidgeting, enclosed/cocoon, itching
>
> *<-> indicates polarity or extremes relating to a theme

The story of the *Rimu* proving echoes information we already have about other conifers used in homeopathy. Rimu is one of New Zealand's tallest indigenous conifers, of the order Pinales. It can grow to around 50 metres tall. Rimu, along with totara, belongs to the family Podocarpaceae. Rimu are found across New Zealand, from Northland to Stewart Island. Rimu trees can live for over a thousand years, but a lifespan of 550 to 650 years is much more common, because strong winds can uproot the tallest, oldest trees. Rimu were the main native tree milled by Europeans during the 20th century for timber to build houses.

The conifer used most often in homeopathy is *Thuja occidentalis*, known also as arbor vitae, or tree of life. Keynote symptoms indicating *Thuja* involve feelings of isolation and alienation. The remedy is associated with strong, rigid beliefs, and with obsessive beliefs, that may relate to religion, health, and diet. *Thuja* is also associated with a sensation of bodily fragility, as if a body is brittle, thin, or delicate. Appearance and self-presentation are important elements linked with *Thuja*. In those for whom *Thuja* is appropriate, attention to detail, and the desire to present a favourable picture, may disguise hidden feelings of guilt. Rigid self-interest can lead to the holding back of information, resulting in manipulation, trickery, and deceit. The remedy *Thuja* is associated with a fear of strangers, dislike of the presence of strangers, or feeling separated from oneself. There may be dreams of death and dying; of one's own death, or the death of others. The theme is a feeling of being divided, with a fixed rigid idea that soul and body are split, or that the mind is separate from the body (Vermeulen & Johnston, 2011, Vol. 3, p. 1270).

The danger of this perception – that the mind is separate from the body – is voiced by the Lorax in Dr Seuss's story as he emerges from a tree stump, shocked and alarmed to find that all the trees have been cut down. In years past, and sadly in the present too, we have cut down trees that sustain entire ecosystems of life on earth, including our own and the life of our planet. Information revealed by our proving of *Rimu* suggests that in cutting down trees we cut ourselves off from an essential part of ourselves: the consciousness we share with each other and all of the Kosmos. Ultimately this leads to a sense of isolation, and disconnection, as the root of our disease.

Throughout history, the concept of the "tree of life" has referred to the interconnection and shared origins of all living things. Tree of life symbolism pervades ancient mythology and many religious traditions. The roots of the tree of life grow deep into the earth below, and the branches reach skyward toward heaven. Conifers are evergreen, representing rebirth and eternal life; traditionally they are well represented in cemeteries. Large conifers, including rimu, are characterised by their longevity; they outlive the mortal lives of humans. These silent sentinels of the forest witness many generations worth of human progress and environmental change. Homeopathy allows access to an imprint of this information: a consciousness retained and stored by the tree.

The ringing cedars

The popular series of non-fiction stories *The Ringing Cedars of Russia* by Vladimir Megre has a similar message (see, for example, book one: Megre, 2008). The books tell the true story of the experiences of the author, a Siberian riverboat trader and entrepreneur, on a journey seeking ancient trees known as ringing cedars. The trees are known to vibrate audibly with strong accumulated energy. On the journey the author encounters Anastasia, a girl who lost her parents very young and grew up under the care of her grandfather and great-grandfather, along with animals in their natural habitat. Anastasia developed extraordinary perceptual abilities and a knowledge of languages and world history she'd never been directly exposed to. She is highly intelligent, with excellent physical health, and seems to draw on the super-conscious; she accesses information unavailable to most of humanity, sharing it with great wisdom.

Homeopathy and allopathy: unable to compete

All the examples given above from the plant order Pinales, reveal the familiar mind–body split belief system that pervades orthodox medicine. A rigid, dualist belief system swept the Western world into a process of mechanisation, materialism, and deforestation. Along the way, doctors who associated in any way with homeopathy were cast out of the system (see Chapter 2).

I've already discussed some of the barriers to homeopathic research being carried out on a large scale (see Chapter 3). In *Divided Legacy*, Coulter considers the economic consequences of the choice of therapeutic method (rationalist vs empiric) when the practice of medicine is also a person's means of earning a living (Coulter, 1982). He warns that socio-economic constraints can influence acceptance or rejection of innovation in medicine, and that this influence occurs irrespective of the science. Choosing the correct homeopathic remedy often involves a time-consuming process. The economic consequences of this fact are accepted as an inherent aspect of the discipline, but this substantially limits the potential for homeopathy to compete with allopathy. Coulter boldly summarises with a confrontational statement: "The tragedy of medical history is that the social, psychological and economic concomitants of medical practice prevent theory from developing along scientific lines."

Tauranga Homeopathy

For me, my immersion for several days in the energy of *Rimu* proved to be a catalyst for personal and collective change. Two of my colleagues from Tauranga attended the same seminar, and at the time we began sharing ideas and visions for the future, feeling drawn together by a common goal. We realised that a collective could achieve much more than an individual. Packing my things on the final day of the seminar, I decided to leave the single silver hoop earring here in the bush where I felt it now belonged. My colleagues and I buried it at the base of the rimu tree from which we had taken material for our proving, and departed in agreement to support our common goal and each other. A fellowship of the ring had formed, and in the statement that had emerged from my proving notes, "Group supports enthusiastic harmony", I took with me the answer to my question.

Six months after that we formed a collective, to be called Tauranga Homeopathy. The power of *Rimu* continued to work with us, as homeopathic remedies can do. We discovered that, much like a spiral does, we needed to start very small, knowing that, in time, we would have the potential to grow, evolve, and develop.

While we were thinking about a potential logo a helpful friend had asked the sensible question "What is homeopathy, and what does it mean to you?" The answer was simple: "It's mind–body–spirit medicine". While considering possible designs, we were drawn to Celtic symbols. An internet search quickly led us to the triple spiral (triskele or triskelion), which looked more like a koru in the early sketches we drew by hand. The koru, based on the shape of an unfurling fern frond, is used in Māori art as a symbol of creation.

The spiral is probably one of the earth's oldest symbols; it has been found in rock carvings thousands of years old on every continent. Dominant meanings of the spiral include action, progress, cycles of revolution, and competition. Three spirals together represent body, mind, and spirit; the familiar equivalent in Christian tradition is the Holy Trinity. They can also refer to levels of development: personal growth, human evolution, and spiritual expansion. A triple spiral usually originates from a common arm, with each spiral expanding outwards. It can also be drawn in the opposite way, with the three spirals meeting at the centre. We chose this latter version: in our logo, three koru extend inwards from a shared outer circle, surrounded by yet another circle. The group of three, surrounded by a ring is also symbolic of us as colleagues, of course.

Figure 4: The Tauranga Homeopathy logo

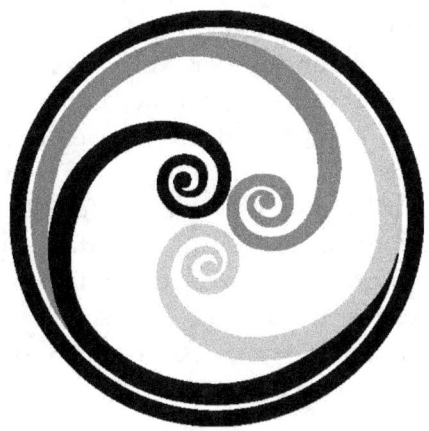

I was ready to devote a greater proportion of my time to homeopathy. When a single clinic room in shared premises became available, Tauranga Homeopathy moved in. At that point, I resolved to leave my medical practice to allow myself more time to work as a homeopath, and to complete this book, promoting a more informed, balanced view of homeopathy. Long-standing loyalties made this a difficult decision. It wasn't easy leaving behind patients and staff I'd come to know, and the secure income my family had relied on. My decision was made easier by the action of *Rimu*. Scholten identifies the conifers as reflecting mainly the themes of the Silver Series or row of elements (Scholten, 2013). In homeopathy, the Silver Series relates directly to creativity, performance, and ideas within art, science, mysticism, and culture. Scholten writes of Podocarpaceae, the family within the plant order of conifers to which rimu belongs, "They are confused about which belief system to choose"(Scholten, 2013, p. 73). The answer to my question had been revealed through my interaction with *Rimu*. I no longer felt confused and was ready to move forward.

When my general practice colleagues asked me what I'd like as a leaving gift, I suggested pounamu jewellery. I knew this was something I wouldn't buy for myself. Pounamu is also referred to as greenstone or New Zealand jade, and was used traditionally for tools and decoration. Expecting to receive a piece of pounamu at my farewell lunch on my last day at the practice, I was unable to speak for a moment when I opened the small box to find a beautiful pair of handmade silver koru earrings, delicately inlaid with pounamu. As my general practice family witnessed my initial surprise followed by obvious excitement and joy, I took the opportunity to share with them the story of *Rimu*, and just a little more information about homeopathy.

Balance and harmony

Nine months has passed since that farewell. I recognise clearly the spiral of life in the slow steady way that progress in my life has occurred since then. This book has evolved to finally reach the stage of completion, to conclude at the "summit", where a wider outlook and a glimpse of the view beyond becomes possible.

For many years I have successfully used homeopathy and orthodox medicine in a complementary way in my clinic, for myself, and for my family: I view them as mutually supportive. I see a future in which many more people could benefit from this dynamic combination. Through sharing some of my personal and professional experiences of the healing effects of homeopathy in this book, my intention is to create a gentle ripple, like that created by a single drop entering the surface of water. The single drop represents both the infinitesimal dose and the manner by which information from a homeopathic substance is dispersed to form a medicine with meaning.

Homeopathy was born during the Age of Enlightenment. As we find ourselves now in the midst of the Age of Information, the time has come for further exploration of the potential of these small powerful catalysts for healing.

My hope is for this book to also become a catalyst for transformation, so that many more people begin to understand how their symptoms, diseases, and suffering similarly convey information; messages from the whole person that must be heard.

GLOSSARY

Acausal: Not following the usual principles of cause and effect, or linear causation. A term used by Jung to describe a relationship characterised by meaning rather than causation. See also **Synchronicity.**

Acute condition: Any illness, injury or trauma of relatively sudden onset with a duration of less than four to six weeks, which would usually result in recovery.

Allopathy: A term used by Samuel Hahnemann to describe orthodox or standard medicine, derived from the Greek words *allo* (other) and *pathos* (suffering or disease). It refers to the treatment of disease with drugs that oppose symptoms in order to remove or suppress them.

Antibodies: Protein molecules produced by blood cells, as part of the immune system response to exposure to a similar substance.

Aphorism: In the context of homeopathy, one of a collection of 291 statements of the principles of homeopathy articulated by Hahnemann in his *Organon of Medicine.*

Aquasol: A minute solid particle dispersed permanently in water.

Bio-medical method: The orthodox medical approach, in which illness is considered to be caused by identifiable factors.

Chi: The vital force or basic life energy that flows through all living things. See also **Traditional Chinese medicine** and **Vital force**.

Chronic: Persisting for a long time. In medicine this usually refers to a period beyond three months.

Classical homeopathy: The method developed by Hahnemann using a single homeopathic substance to treat the whole person (mental, emotional, and physical symptoms), rather than the disease. See also **Constitutional homeopathy**.

Colloid: A non-crystalline substance in which particles of one substance are dispersed through a second substance and are thereafter unable to be separated out by filtering or centrifuging.

Constitutional homeopathy: Another way of describing **Classical homeopathy**, treating the whole person (mental, emotional, and physical symptoms), rather than the disease.

Double blind: Denoting an experiment or procedure in which neither the researcher nor the subject knows whether the subject has received an intervention/treatment or placebo.

Dualism: The conceptual separation of something into two contrasting or opposing parts, thereby creating a division.

Empiricism: The idea that knowledge originates from observation and experience.

Epitaxy: The transfer of information without matter, resulting in the imprinting of one structure onto another.

Genus epidemicus: A single remedy that homeopaths find to be effective for multiple sufferers of a particular epidemic.

Holarchy: Koestler's term for a natural hierarchy of increasing wholeness (the whole of one level becomes a part of the whole of the next level). See also **Holon**.

Holon: Koestler's term for any entity that is itself a whole and simultaneously a part of some other whole. See also **Holarchy**.

Individualisation: The concept of choosing an exact homeopathic remedy for a particular person, to be given at the right time, in the right potency or dose.

Infinitesimal dose: An extremely small dose mathematically approaching zero.

Kosmos: Wilber's conceptualisation of everything in the universe, comprising elements of matter, life, mind, and spirit.

Law of Similars: The principle on which homeopathy is based, that a homeopathic remedy that most closely matches a person's symptoms can have a healing or curative effect.

Lebenswelt: life-world. Husserl's concept to describe a multidimensional experienced reality, of which the scientific world is just one part.

Materia medica: a book indexed by remedy, describing symptoms noted in provings, accidental poisonings and successfully "cured" cases. See also **Repertory**.

Miasm: A concept first used by Hahnemann to describe characteristics of three common diseases of his time (syphilis, gonorrhoea, and scabies). Used by homeopaths more recently to describe predisposing patterns of disease expression.

Mindfulness: A state of non-judgemental awareness of the present moment allowing acceptance of thoughts, feelings, and physical sensations.

Minimum dose: A homeopathic remedy given in the lowest dose that is effective without producing unwanted adverse effects.

Nocebo effect: A harmful or negative effect experienced by a patient after receiving an inactive substance or therapeutic intervention. See also **Placebo**.

Nosode: A homeopathic remedy made from disease matter that has undergone potentisation so that no molecule of the original disease substance is present.

Pilule: A miniature pill, usually made of sugar (sucrose), which can be medicated with a homeopathic solution. Some suppliers use milk sugar (lactose).

Placebo: An inactive substance given or procedure undertaken that has no known intrinsic therapeutic value.

Potentisation: The process of serial dilution and succussion of a solution containing a substance, as described by Hahnemann, used to create a homeopathic remedy.

Prana: The universal energy or life force that maintains life and health; it is breathed in and out. See also **Chi** and **Vital force**.

Prognosis: A forecast or prediction of the probable course and outcome of a disorder.

Prophylaxis: Intervention or treatment used for the prevention of disease.

Proving: A system of experimentation whereby a homeopathic substance is administered to a group of volunteers who record all their symptoms, to discover the effects and properties of the substance.

Psychosomatic: Denoting physical symptoms or illness caused by emotional or psychological factors.

Randomised control trial (RCT): A form of research comparing results from a group of patients who receive a treatment with another "control" group who do not receive treatment, where randomisation is used to allocate patients to either group.

Rationalism: The idea that knowledge is intellectual, and therefore is acquired by logical deduction rather than through observation, sensory perception, and experience.

Remedy: Homeopathic medicine or preparation.

Repertorisation: The process of translating a patient's characteristic symptoms into similar symptoms, known as rubrics. See also **Repertory**.

Repertory: a book indexed by symptoms, listing particular remedies known to cause or reproduce a specific symptom. See also **Repertorisation** and **Materia medica**.

Sarcode: A homeopathic remedy made from healthy human or animal tissue or secretions. **Potentisation** means no molecule of the original substance is present in the remedy.

Serial dilution: A method of stepwise dilution used to reduce the concentration of a solution by the same amount at each step.

Simillimum: The homeopathic substance capable of causing symptoms most similar to the totality of symptoms (mental, emotional, and physical) expressed by a person being treated.

Somatisation: The expression of psychological stress as physical symptoms.

Strange, rare, or peculiar (SRP) symptoms: Uncommon symptoms associated with a patient or a remedy, often without any logical or rational explanation, that help individualise a case (or remedy).

Succussion: The process of vigorous shaking used in **Potentisation** whereby a vial of solution is knocked multiple times against a firm surface.

Synchronicity: A word used by Jung to describe cases of meaningful coincidence or an association of events that are connected but not causally linked. See also **Acausal**.

Tao: A word used within Chinese philosophy to describe the absolute reality or principle underlying the natural universe, which can be considered undefinable. See also **Synchronicity**.

Totality of Symptoms: A term used first by Hahnemann in his *Organon of Medicine* to refer to all the symptoms of a case that can be combined into a coherent consistent individualised whole indicating the simillimum. See also **Simillimum**.

Traditional Chinese medicine (TCM): An ancient Chinese system of healing using a number of interventions, including acupuncture, herbal remedies, dietary changes, massage, and exercise to treat illnesses, which are viewed as imbalances or disharmony.

Trituration: The process of grinding a substance with an inactive powder to make the substance soluble. Also "A dry method of potentising medicinal substances whereby the substance is finely ground in a mortar with a certain proportion of milk sugar , thereby progressively attenuating it" (Hogeland & Schriebman, 2008, p. V).

Ultramolecular dilution: see **Infinitesimal dose**.

Vital force: Hahnemann's term for the life force or energy that animates living organisms, disturbances of which are expressed as symptoms or disease. See also **Chi**.

REFERENCES

Anyan, S. (2012, July). Homeopathy – trick or treatment? *North and South*, 42–43.

Benveniste, J., Arnoux, B., & Hadji, L. (1992). Highly dilute antigen increases coronary flow of isolated heart from immunised guinea-pigs. *FASEB Journal, 6*, A1610.

Benveniste, J., Aissa, J., Litime, M. H., Tsaegaca, G. T., & Thomas, Y. (1994). Transfer of the molecular signal by electronic amplification. *FASEB Journal, 8*(4), A2304.

Brennan, B. A. (1988). *Hands of light: A guide to healing through the human energy field.* New York, NY: Bantam Books.

Broom, B. (1997). *Somatic illness and the patient's other story: A practical integrative mind/body approach to disease for doctors and psychotherapists.* London: Free Association Books.

Broom, B. (2007). *Meaning-full disease: How personal experience and meanings cause and maintain physical illness.* London: Karnac Books.

Buettner, C., Kroenke, C., Phillips, R. S., Davis, R. B., Eisenberg, D. M., & Holmes, M. D. (2006). Correlates of use of different types of complementary and alternative medicine by breast cancer survivors in the nurses' health study. *Breast Cancer Research and Treatment, 100*(2), 219–227.

Chopra, D. (2003). *Synchro-destiny: Harnessing the infinite power of coincidence to create miracles.* London: Rider.

Coulter, H. L. (1982). *Divided legacy: The conflict between homeopathy and the American Medical Association* (Vol. 3) (2nd ed.). Washington, DC: Center for Empirical Medicine.

Coulter, H. L. (1994). *Divided legacy: The patterns emerge, Hippocrates to Paracelsis* (Vol. 1). Washington, DC: Center for Empirical Medicine. (Original work published 1975)

Coulter, I. & Willis, E. (2004). The rise and rise of complementary and alternative medicine: a sociological perspective. *Medical Journal of Australia 180*(11), 587–589.

Cristea, A., Nicula, S., & Darie, V. (1997). Pharmacodynamic effects of very high dilutions of belladonna on isolated rat duodenum. In M. Bastide (Ed.), *Signals and Images* (pp. 161–170). Dordrecht: Springer.

Davenas, E., Beauvais, F., Amara, J., Oberbaum, M., Robinzon, B., Miadonna, A., Tedeschi, A., Pomeranz, B., Fortner, P., Belon, P., et al. (1988). Human basophil degranulation triggered by very dilute antiserum against IgE. *Nature, 333*(6176), 816–818.

Deveugele, M., Derese, A., van den Brink-Muinen, A., Bensing, J., & De Maeseneer, J. (2002). Consultation length in general practice: cross sectional study in six European countries. *British Medical Journal 325*, 472.

Emoto, M. (2005). *The true power of water: Healing and discovering ourselves*. Hillsboro, OR: Beyond Words Publishing.

Hahnemann, S. (2004). *Organon of medicine* (6th ed.). New Delhi: B. Jain. (Original work published 1921)

Harris, R. (2007). *The happiness trap: Stop struggling and start living*. China: Exisle.

Hogeland, A. & Schriebman, J. (2008). *The trituration handbook: Into the heart of homeopathy*. El Cerrito, CA: Homeopathy West.

Ho, M.-W. (2011). Quantum Coherent Water, Non-thermal EMF Effects, and Homeopathy, Institute of Science in Society.

Hughes, B. (2010). *The hemlock cup: Socrates, Athens and the search for the good life.* New York, NY: Random House.

Jung, C. G. (1960). *Synchronicity: An acausal connecting principle. From Vol. 8 of the collected works of C. G. Jung.* Princeton, NJ: Princeton University Press.

Kelly, R. (2008). *The human antenna: Reading the language of the universe in the songs of our cells.* Santa Rosa, CA: Energy Psychology Press.

Kelly, R. (2011). *The human hologram: Living your life in harmony with the unified field.* Santa Rosa, CA: Energy Psychology Press.

Kent, J. T. (1921). Kent's repertory (6th ed.). New Delhi: B. Jain.

Kooreman, P. & Baars, E. (2012). Patients whose GP knows complementary medicine tend to have lower costs and live longer. *European Journal of Health Economics 13*(6), 769–776.

Lipton, B. H. (2008). *The biology of belief: Unleashing the power of consciousness, matter & miracles.* United States: Hay House.

Lipton, B. H. & Bhaerman, S. (2009). *Spontaneous evolution: Our positive future and a way to get there from here.* United States: Hay House.

McTaggart, L. (2001). *The field: The quest for the secret force of the universe.* London: Element.

Megre, V. (2008). *Anastasia (The ringing cedars series, Book One)* (2nd revised ed.). United States: Ringing Cedar Press.

Millman, D. (1985). *Way of the peaceful warrior: A book that changes lives.* Timburon, CA: H. J. Kramer.

Ministerial Advisory Committee of Complementary and Alternative Health. (2007). *CAM Consumers.* Wellington: Ministry of Health.

Poynton, L., Dowell, A., Dew, K., & Egan, T. (2006). General practitioners' attitudes towards (and use of) complementary and alternative medicine: a New Zealand nationwide survey. *New Zealand Medical Journal 119*(1247), 35–44.

Rey, L. (2003). "Thermoluminescence of ultra-high dilutions of lithium chloride and sodium chloride." PhysicaA **323**: 67-74.

Ross, A. C. G. (1982). *Homoeopathy: An introductory guide.* Wellingborough: Thorston.

Roy, R., Tiller, W. A., Bell, I., Hoover, M. R. (2005). The structure of liquid water; novel insights from materials research; potential relevance to homeopathy. *Materials Research Innovations,* 9-4, 1433-075X.

Scholten, J. (2002). *Homoeopathy and the elements.* Utrecht: Stichting Alonnissos.

Scholten, J (2005). *Secret lanthanides.* Utrecht: Stichting Alonnissos.

Scholten, J. (2013). *Wonderful plants.* Utrecht: Stichting Alonnissos.

Sheldrake, R. (1987). *A new science of life: The hypothesis of formative causation.* London: Paladin.

Sheldrake, R. (2003). *The sense of being stared at.* London: Arrow Books.

Sheldrake, R. (2011). *Dogs that know when their owners are coming home: And other unexplained powers of animals.* London: Arrow Books.

Tiller, W. (2006). "On chemical medicine, thermodynamics, and homeopathy." J Altern Complement Med **12**(7): 685-93.

Vermeulen, F. & Johnston, L. (2011). *Plants: Homeopathic and medicinal uses from a botanical family perspective* (Vols. 1–4). Glasgow: Saltire Books.

Virtue, D. (1997). *The Lightworker's way: Awakening your spiritual power to know and heal.* United States: Hay House.

Watson, L. (1979). *Lifetide: The biology of unconscious.* New York, NY: Simon & Schuster.

Whitmont, E. (1986). *Psyche and substance: Essays on homeopathy in the light of Jungian Psychology.* New Delhi: Indian Books & Periodicals Syndicate.

Wilber, K. (2000). *A brief history of everything* (2nd ed.). Boston, MA: Shambhala.

Winston, J. (1999). *The faces of homoeopathy: An illustrated history of the first 200 years.* Wellington: Great Auk Publishing.

World Health Organization (2002). World Health Organization (2002) Safety of Medicines. A guide to detecting and reporting adverse drug reactions: Why health professionals need to take action. Geneva, WHO.

World Health Organization (2015). Antimicrobial resistance, WHO.

Youngson, R. (2012). *Time to care: How to love your patients and your job.* Raglan: Rebelheart Publishers.

FURTHER INFORMATION AVAILABLE ONLINE

http://www.britishhomeopathic.org
(British Homeopathic Association)

http://www.facultyofhomeopathy.org
(United Kingdom Faculty of Homeopathy)

http://www.homeopathy.co.nz
(New Zealand Council of Homeopaths)

http://homeopathy.ac.nz
(New Zealand Homeopathic Society)

https://www.homeopathy.org
(North American Society of Homeopaths)

http://www.hpus.com
(Homœopathic Pharmacopœia of the United States)

INDEX